365 DAYS
OF
ESSENTIAL OILS

365 Essential Oils Recipes for 365 Days

White Lemon

365 Days of Essential Oils

Disclaimer

ISBN-13: 978-1539929468

Contents

Introduction xiii

January

Facial Oil for Dehydrated Skin 3
Rose Moisturizer 3
Moisturizing Lip Balm... 3
Invigorating Shower Gel 4
Healing Balm for Dry Hands 4
Re-Energizing Aroma Therapy Diffuser Blend.. 4
Winter Blend for the Diffuser 4
Soothing Bath Oil 5
Easy Drawer Fresheners.. 5
Lemon Wood Polish 5
Hair Oil 5
Massage Oil for Nails... 6
Room Freshener 6
Sweet and Nutty Movie Night Snack Mix 6
Oatmeal Raisin Bars 7
Kids' Play Dough 7
Exotic Citrus Perfume.. 7
Invigorating Body Scrub 8
Foaming Skin Cleanser 8
Cough Syrup 8
Hair Gel.. 8
Orange Soap Bars 9
Rainbow Soap Bars 9
Lemon Facial Scrub 9
Sore Muscle Massage Oil.. 10
Compress for Fevers.. 10
Fever Socks 10
Sore Throat Gargle.. 10
Sinus Steam... 11
Essential Oil Cold Sore Treatment 11
Sinus-Ease Humidifier Blend 11
Swollen Ankle Massage Oil.. 11
How to Have Your Own Essential Oils Spa Party................................... 12

February

Valentine's Day Scent for Women..17
Valentine's Day Scent for Men...17
Luxurious Cleanser..17
Eye Cream...17
Shaving Cream...18
Neck Cream...18
Aftershave...19
Elbow Cream...19
Luscious, Kissable Lip Balm...19
Hot and Spicy Lip Balm...20
Chicken Alfredo...20
Baked Ham Glaze...20
Puffy Eyes Blend..21
Refreshing Body Scrub..21
Body Butter...21
Bath Melts..22
Sweet-Smelling Pendant..22
Lavender Bars..22
Copycat Burt's Bees Lip Balm..23
Body Wash..23
Orange Body Spray...23
Patchouli Body Spray..24
Home-Made Dish Soap..24
All-Purpose Cleaner..24
Dryer Sheets...24
Pet Shampoo...25
Rub for Swollen Feet..25
Bath Oil to Relieve Exhaustion...25
Dry Shampoo..26
Make Your Own Facial Clay Masks..**26**

March

Egyptian Goddess Perfume..29
Cleansing Body Scrub..29
Facial Toner...29
Cleansing Mask..29
Refreshing Foot Bath..30
Acne Treatment...30
Hand Treatment...30
Face Gel Acne Blend...30

Face Gel Dry Skin Blend 31
Face Gel Problem Skin Blend 31
Shower Gel 31
Puffy Eye Tonic 32
All Over Moisturizer 32
Anti-Aging Mask 32
Rose Moisturizer 33
Relaxation Perfume 33
Fruit Salsa 33
Cinnamon Chips 33
Garden Smoothie 34
Anti-Wrinkle Oil 34
Pine Floor Cleaner 34
Carpet Deodorizer 34
Citrus Dishwashing Liquid 35
Oven Cleaner 35
Flea Repellant 35
Stretch Mark Formula 36
Alopecia Shampoo 36
Hair Loss Lotion 36
Diaper Rash Treatment 36
Cough Solution for Babies and Children 37
Poise Perfume 37
How to Make Your Own Perfumes Using Essential Oils **38**

April

Cough Drops 41
Lemongrass Scrub 41
Sensitive Skin Clay Mask 41
Exfoliating Body Scrub 41
Doggie Flea Collar 1 42
Doggie Flea Collar 2 42
Heartburn Relief 42
Baby Massage Oil 43
Foamy Carpet Shampoo 43
Toilet Bowl Cleaner 43
Toothpaste 43
Garlic and Herb Chicken 44
Cilantro Salad Dressing 44
Yogurt Dip 44
Air Freshener 45
Citrus Mint Diffuser Blend 45

Sleepy Time Pillow Spray 45
Backache Massage Oil 1 45
Backache Massage Oil 2 46
Bubble Gum/Mint Lip Balm 46
Gel Air Freshener 46
Detoxifying Hair Mask 47
Pimple Relief 47
Insect Repellent 47
Allergy Relief 48
Diaper Rash Relief 48
Washing Machine Freshener 48
Canker Sore Treatment 49
Sweet-Smelling Wax Melts 49
Ear Infection Remedy 49
House Cleaning with Essential Oils **50**

May

Self-Confidence Perfume 53
Body Scrub 53
Skin Revitalizing Mask 53
Wrinkle Cream 53
Hand Cream for Mom 54
Concentration Diffusion Blend 54
Pick-Me-Up Diffusion Blend 54
Kitchen Aroma Therapy 54
Revitalizing Bath Oil 55
Bath Fizzies 55
Air Spray 55
Easy Liquid Soap 55
Refreshing Body Oil 56
Kitchen Cleaner 56
Handbag Freshener 56
Man Bag Freshener 56
Drawer Freshener 57
Kitchen Soap 57
Jet Lag Swollen Ankle Formula 57
Travel Sickness Blend 57
Insect Repellent 58
Ylang Ylang Hair Oil 58
Cuticle Soak 58
Essential Oil Candies 58
Chocolate Mint Bars 59

Springtime Chicken Bake 59
Hot Toddy for Adults...59
Dog Flea Shampoo 60
Doggie Arthritis Treatment...60
Pregnancy Constipation Formula 60
Hair Conditioning Treatment for Baldness 60
Using Aroma Therapy Diffusers **61**

June

Aromatherapy Bath Salts 65
Chicken Taquitos..65
Cream Deodorant 65
Acne Clay Mask..66
Stick Deodorant..66
Lavender Skin Tonic 66
Rose Bath Gel 66
Foamy Bath Oil 67
Sore Foot Soak 67
Athlete's Foot Soak 67
Hand Soap 68
Brush-In Hair Scent 68
After-Sun Skin Re-Hydrator 68
Focus Your Mind Room Spritz 68
Feta Dip 69
Lavender Rose Solid Perfume..69
Wart Treatment 69
Bruise Treatment..69
Lavender Infused Lemonade 70
Carpet Freshener 70
Citrus Mint Room Spray 70
Rheumatism Rub..70
Sore Muscle Massage Oil 1 71
Sore Muscle Massage Oil 2 71
Colored Bath Salts..71
Body Dusting Powder 71
Softening Lip Balm...72
Almond/Oatmeal Facial Scrub 72
Super-Insect Repellent 72
Summer Perfume 73
Tips for Cooking with Essential Oils..**74**

July

After-Sun Aloe Vera Gel 77
Soothing Sunburn Lotion 77
Sunscreen Lotion Bars 77
Cherry Lemonade 78
Peppermint Iced Tea 78
Happiness Perfume 78
Coconut Body Scrub 78
Mature Skin Clay Mask 79
Relaxation Diffuser Blend 79
Brain Power Diffuser Blend 79
Bath Fizz 79
Conditioning Hair Oil 80
Scented Foot Powder 80
Foot Bath 80
Clay Mask for Normal Skin 81
Dry Skin Clay Facial Mask 81
Oily Skin Clay Facial Mask 81
Sunscreen Bar 81
Insect Repellent Bar 82
Uplifting Perfume 82
Intestinal Ailment Blend 82
Multi-Purpose Cleaner 83
Flea and Tick Repellent 83
Wrinkle Cream 83
Glowing Skin Exfoliate 83
Romantic Massage Oil 84
Sore Joint Oil 84
Air Freshening Spray 84
Carpet Freshener 84
Pet Odor Diffuser Blend 85
Citrus Popsicles 85
Make Solid Perfume with Essential Oils **86**

August

Slow Cooker Meatballs 89
Home-Made Pasta Sauce 89
Shower Gel 89
Mood Enhancing Perfume 90
Athlete's Foot/Ringworm Treatment 90
Burn Treatment 90

Bed-Time Aroma Therapy 90

Facial Cleanser 91

Foaming Facial Cleanser 91

Shaving Cream 91

Aftershave 92

Elbow Cream 92

Eye Tonic 92

Aloe Vera Face Gel for Dry Skin 93

Aloe Vera Face Gel for Problem Skin 93

Aloe Vera Face Gel for Acne 93

Acne Treatment 93

Morning Shower Gel 94

Soft Lips Balm 94

Hand Oil 94

Neck Cream 95

Acne Face Mask 95

Peaceful Perfume 95

Family Room Diffuser Blend 95

Lavender Bath Fizz 96

Dandruff Hair Oil 96

Revitalizing Facial Mask 96

Citrus Room Spritz 96

Citrus Body Spray 97

Sea Salt Facial Scrub 97

Temple Massage Oil 97

Essential Oils and Pregnancy..**98**

September

Disinfecting Bathroom Diffuser Blend 101

Rose Bath Fizz 101

Scalp Massage Oil 101

Essential Oil Shampoo 101

Anti-Fungal Foot Soak 102

Purifying Facial Mask 102

Citrus Bathroom Spray 102

Sore Muscle Rub 102

Headache Rub 103

Kids' Aroma Therapy for Colds 103

Exfoliating Foot Scrub 103

Relaxing Massage Oil 103

Woodsy Air Freshener 104

Air Purifying Aroma Therapy 104

Chicken Noodle Soup..104
Cinnamon Milk...105
Fruit Dip..105
Citrus Floor Cleaner...105
Kitchen Pest Control...105
Dog Earwax Treatment...106
Kitty Flea Collar..106
Hair Loss Oil Treatment...106
Jasmine Perfume..106
Woodsy Perfume..107
Rose Moisturizer..107
Lavender Lip Balm...107
Citrus Shower Gel..107
Lavender Bubble Bath..108
Corn and Callus Relief...108
Minty-Fresh Body Powder..108
Essential Oils and Babies..109

October

Cinnamon Candy Apples 113
Acne Steam Bath..113
Foot Deodorizer Powder 113
Skin Care Massage Oil 114
Simple Lip Balm 114
Love and Devotion Perfume 114
Relaxation Perfume...114
Sugar Scrub Cubes...115
Cranberry Lip Balm..115
Cranberry Hair Rinse...115
Cinnamon Spice Lip Gloss...116
Anti-Wrinkle Serum 116
Anti-Wrinkle Facial Mask...116
Cranberry Face Wash...116
Wrinkle Cream...117
Honey Cashew Candy 117
Cinnamon Candy Popcorn Balls..117
Peppermint Foot Cream..118
Romantic Lubricant..118
Mystical Body Spray...118
Eastern Essence Perfume..118
Citrus Scrub 119
Cinnamon/Orange Diffuser Blend..119

Excitement Perfume 119
Ginger Skin Scrub 119
Orange/Clove Soap 120
Lift Me Up Perfume 120
Cinnamon Hot Chocolate 120
Cinnamon Orange Diffuser Blend 121
Lavender Body Spray 121
Pumpkin Spice Soap 121
How to Give an Essential Oil Hand Massage **122**

November

Pumpkin Pie Spice Oil 125
Pumpkin Spice Diffuser Blend 125
Allergy Formula 125
Hairspray 125
Spirit-Lifting Perfume 126
Vapor Rub 126
Honey Lotion Bars 126
Happiness Perfume 126
Peppermint Body Butter 127
Spicy Air Freshener 127
Pumpkin Soup 127
Pumpkin Bread 128
Bronzing Body Butter 128
Happiness Perfume 128
Holiday Spice Room Spray 129
Citrus Mint Layered Soap 129
Softening Lip Balm 129
Cinnamon Spice Tea 130
Minty Bath Salts 130
Healing Gel for Rashes 130
Light and Fresh Diffuser Blend 131
Soothing Bath Oil 131
Foaming Hand Soap 131
Peppermint Skin Toner 131
Be Alert Diffuser Blend 132
Cold and Flu Steam 132
Cough Relief 132
Invigorating Bath Oil 132
Coconut Body Scrub 133
Winter Warmth Perfume 133
The Benefits of Using Essential Oils **134**

December

Slow Cooker Turkey Meatballs with Cranberry/BBQ Sauce 137
Seasonal Diffuser Blend 137
Citrus and Spice Hot Cider... 137
Gingerbread Man Mini Soap 138
Scented Holiday Ornaments.. 138
Sweet Cranberry Sauce 138
Holiday Perfume 139
Star Soap 139
Stovetop Kitchen Freshener 139
Holiday Bath Salts 140
Orange/Cinnamon Facial Scrub 140
Peppermint Lip Balm... 140
Holiday Diffuser Blend 141
Baked Ham with Glaze 141
Orange Clove Closet Freshener.. 141
Candy Cane Drawer Freshener 142
Scar Treatment 142
Invigorating Massage Oil.. 142
Holiday Air Spray 142
Holiday Air Spray 2 143
Lavender Face Lotion.. 143
Candy Cane Skin Toner 143
Facial Moisturizer... 144
Holiday Hot Chocolate Gift Pack... 144
Holiday Turkey 144
Boxing Day Leftover Turkey Stir-Fry 145
Minty Fresh Floor Cleaner 145
Sink Stain Remover 145
Kitchen Wipes... 146
Moisturizing Facial Mask 146
New Year's Eve Perfume.. 146
Conclusion... **147**

Bonus Essential Oils 149

*1*NTRODUCTION

When it comes to caring for yourself, your family, and your home, you want to use products that are safe and healthy. Unfortunately, many of the products you buy for cleaning, skin care, hair care, etc. are loaded with chemicals, and may not actually be as safe to use as you may think. But, there is a way that you can get around this. You can make your own products, quickly and easily, and in most cases you only need a few ingredients. The key ingredients in these recipes are essential oils. In this book, you will find 365 awesome recipes that use essential oils, for everything from hair care to pet care to house cleaning to baby care and even food recipes. Interspersed throughout this book are also how-to articles so you will be able to easily use essential oils in your everyday life.

January

Christmas is over, and now the winter blahs are beginning to set in. It is also cold and flu season, so in addition to feeling down, a lot of people are feeling downright sick. Luckily, there are all kinds of treatments for just about any ailment that use essential oils. Whether you just want something to help you perk up on a dark, dreary winter day, or something to help treat a cold or even chapped lips, you will find what you need right here.

Facial Oil for Dehydrated Skin

Materials

4 tablespoons avocado oil
2 tablespoon jojoba oil
2 tablespoon rosehip oil
6 drops Jasmine
4 drops Sandalwood

6 drops Ylang Ylang
Dark colored glass bottle
Funnel
Label and marker

Directions

Combine avocado oil, jojoba oil, and rosehip oil and pour into glass bottle through a funnel. Add oils and shake. Remember to shake before each use to mix ingredients. Label the bottle, including the date made.

Rose Moisturizer
January 2

Materials

1 tablespoon shredded or grated beeswax
¼ cup jojoba oil
¼ cup apricot kernel oil

1 tsp rosehip oil
1 tbsp rosewater
8 drops rose essential oil

Directions

Combine beeswax, jojoba oil and apricot kernel oil in a glass Pyrex jar. Set the jar in a frying pan with simmering water, and let ingredients melt together. Place rosewater in another jar, and put this jar in another frying pan with simmering water. When ingredients in the first jar are combined, add the rosehip oil and mix well. Slowly add rosewater with a dropper, removing oil mixture from heat when 1 tbsp of rosewater has been added. Keep adding rosewater, mixing with a whisk. When it gets thick, add rose essential oil. Pour mixture into jars, cover, and label with the date.

Moisturizing Lip Balm
January 3

Materials

4 tsp grated beeswax or beeswax pellets
2 tsp shea butter
8 tbsp apricot oil

2 tsp carrot-infused oil
12 drops mint essential oil
Lip balm tubes or pots

Directions

In a double boiler over medium heat, combine beeswax, apricot oil, and shea butter. When ingredients have melted together, add carrot-infused oil, mixing well. Add mint essential oil as mixture cools. Pour into lip balm tubes or pots, and label with the date.

Invigorating Shower Gel

Materials

2C shower gel base
20 drops geranium essential oil
16 drops rosemary essential oil

20 drops bergamot essential oil
8 drops juniper essential oil

Directions

Combine shower gel base with essential oils, adding the oils one drop at a time and mixing as you work. Mix slowly to avoid a lot of bubbles in the mixture. Once everything is well-mixed, pour into a pump bottle. Label with the date.

Healing Balm for Dry Hands

January 5

Materials

10 tbsp shea butter
6 tbsp jojoba oil
4 tbsp shredded beeswax
2 tbsp avocado oil

4 tbsp rice bran oil
10 drops each pink grapefruit, lemon, and orange essential oils

Directions

Combine beeswax, jojoba oil, shea butter, rice bran oil, and avocado oil in a double boiler. Stir until ingredients are melted and well-mixed. Remove from heat, continuing to stir. Add scents before mixture begins to thicken, stirring to mix. Pour into jars, cover, and label with the date. Allow mixture to sit overnight, and then use two or more times daily for soft hands.

Re-Energizing Aroma Therapy Diffuser Blend

January 6

Materials

6 drops peppermint essential oil
4 drops cedar wood essential oil

2 drops pine essential oil

Directions

Add all essential oils to a diffuser. Follow the instructions from the "How to Use a Diffuser" section of this book.

Winter Blend for the Diffuser

January 7

Materials

3 drops clove essential oil
3 drops ginger essential oil

5 drops cinnamon essential oil

Directions

Add all essential oils to a diffuser. Follow the instructions from the "How to Use a Diffuser" section of this book.

Soothing Bath Oil   January 8

Materials

7 drops lavender oil
5 drops rose oil
5 drops lemon balm

½ C carrier oil (rice bran oil, coconut oil, etc.)

Directions

Mix all ingredients together. Place into a clean jar, and label with the date. Use mixture in the bath, or after bathing, massage this oil into your skin.

Easy Drawer Fresheners   January 9

Materials

Orange essential oil
Lemon essential oil
Lavender essential oil

Rose essential oil
Cotton balls

Directions

Put a couple of drops of essential oils onto cotton balls. Use single oils, or combine for your own signature scent. Experiment with other oils for more scents to freshen all of your drawers.

Lemon Wood Polish   January 10

Materials

1 tsp lemon essential oil

1 C olive oil

Directions

Mix in a spray bottle. Apply to wood furniture, and wipe with a soft cloth.

Hair Oil   January 11

Materials

½ ounce carrier oil
2 drops clary sage oil
2 drops rosemary oil

2 drops jasmine absolute oil
2 drops lavender oil

Directions

Combine all ingredients in a dark glass bottle. Shake well. Refrigerate if you are not going to use it right away.

Massage Oil for Nails   January 12

Materials

4 ml rice bran oil
2 drops lemon oil
2 drops lavender oil

2 drops tea tree oil
2 drops benzoin absolute resin
1 vitamin E capsule

Directions

Combine materials into a small glass jar and blend well. Use two drops on each fingernail and toenail, and massage into the nails. You can also use this as a hand massage oil, doubling the amount that you would use on a single nail.

Room Freshener   January 13

Materials

½ C pure distilled water
50 drops lime essential oil
25 drops tangerine essential oil

40 drops bergamot essential oil
10 drops petitgrain essential oil
1 tsp emulsifier

Directions

Mix oils and emulsifier. Add distilled water, and pour mixture into a spray bottle. Mixture may be cloudy, but this is okay. Shake before using.

Sweet and Nutty Movie Night Snack Mix   January 14

Materials

3 C whole, raw nuts
1/3 C agave nectar

2 drops cinnamon essential oil
1 tbsp butter

Directions

Melt butter in a saucepan over medium heat. Add nuts and agave nectar, and cook for 10-15 minutes, stirring constantly to keep mixture from burning and sticking to the pot. When there is a scent from the cooked nuts, remove from heat, and add cinnamon oil, stirring to coat. Place coated nuts on parchment paper until cooled, either separated or in clusters.

*O*ATMEAL RAISIN BARS

Materials

1C softened butter
1 ½ C agave nectar
2 eggs
1 tsp vanilla
1C raisins
1 ¾ C whole oat flour

1 tsp baking soda
½ tsp salt
3C rolled oats
1 C chocolate chips
1-2 drops young living cinnamon bark
essential oil

Directions

Cream butter and agave nectar until creamy. Add eggs, vanilla, and essential oil, beating well. Add flour, soda, and sale, beating well. Add oats, raisins, and chocolate chips, stirring to blend. Spread mixture onto a 9"X13" ungreased baking pan. Bake at 350 degrees for 30-35 minutes. Cut into bars.

*K*IDS' PLAY DOUGH

Materials

1 C flour
½ C salt
2 tsp cream of tartar
1 C water

1 ½ tbsp. olive oil or other cooking oil
Food coloring
5-10 drops of your choice of essential oils
for scents

Directions

Combine flour, salt, and cream of tartar in a saucepan. Add oil, water, and food coloring, and blend until smooth. Heat on medium-low, stirring until a ball is formed. Once it is at a play-dough consistency, remove from heat and knead in your favorite essential oils. Store in the fridge in an air-tight container.

*E*XOTIC CITRUS PERFUME

Materials

1 drop frankincense essential oil
2 drops juniper essential oil
5 drops orange essential oil

1 tsp carrier oil (jojoba or almond oil)
1 tsp vodka or other clear alcohol

Directions

Combine carrier oil and alcohol into the bottle that will hold your perfume. Add essential oils, one drop at a time, shaking after the addition of each drop. Cap bottle and store in a cool, dark place for about two weeks. Shake bottle three times daily. Perfume will last longer when stored in the fridge.

*I*NVIGORATING BODY SCRUB **January 18**

Materials

3-4 drops peppermint essential oil
5 tbsp coarse sea salt

½ tsp carrier oil (rice bran, grapeseed, etc.)
Water

Directions

Mix peppermint oil and sea salt, then add carrier oil. Add a bit of water to make the mixture moist. Massage into skin and rinse.

*F*OAMING SKIN CLEANSER **January 19**

Materials

4 tbsp castile or other liquid soap base
3 tsp avocado oil
4 drops lemon essential oil

4 drops orange essential oil
4 drops grapefruit essential

Directions

Combine in a bottle and shake well. Label with date. Remember to shake up the ingredients before each use.

*C*OUGH SYRUP **January 20**

Materials

½ C raw honey
4-5 drops cinnamon essential oil

1 tsp ginger

Directions

Combine all ingredients and store in a dark bottle in the fridge. Label with the date. Take one teaspoon of the mixture at a time, about 3-4 times daily to alleviate cold symptoms.

*H*AIR GEL **January 21**

Materials

3-4 C golden flax seeds
1 gallon distilled water
2 tbsp liquid aloe vera
2 vitamin E capsules
3-4 drops peppermint essential oil

Directions

Combine flax seeds and distilled water in a double boiler. Cook over medium heat until mixture turns into a slimy jelly. Stir in aloe vera, liquid from vitamin E capsules, and peppermint oil. Cool, and strain out the flax seeds. Store in the fridge in jars.

ORANGE SOAP BARS   January 22

Materials

Glycerin soap base
5-6 drops food grade orange color
5-10 drops orange essential oil

1 tbsp liquid aloe vera
Soap bar mold (4 3-ounce bars per mold)

Directions

In a double boiler, melt glycerin soap base over medium heat. Add color, essential oil, and aloe vera, and pour into molds. Let set for a couple of hours, remove from molds, and wrap with waxed paper or parchment paper.

RAINBOW SOAP BARS   January 22

Materials

Glycerin soap base
Orange, red, yellow, green, blue, purple, pink food grade color

5-10 drops of the essential oil of your choice
Bread loaf pan

Directions

Melt 3 ounces of glycerin soap base in a double boiler. Add one of the colors, and a couple of drops of essential oil. Pour into bread loaf pan, and let cool. Repeat process for all of the colors, until you have layered all of the colors. Once cool, remove from loaf pan and cut into slices for rainbow soap bars.

LEMON FACIAL SCRUB   January 23

Materials

½ C Coarse sea salt or sugar
4-5 drops lemon essential oil

1 tsp liquid aloe vera

Directions

Combine all ingredients. Rub into face, being careful on any areas where the skin is sensitive. Rinse with cool water.

Sore Muscle Massage Oil

Materials

1 ounce carrier oil (rice bran, grapeseed, etc.)

5-6 drops lavender oil

Directions

Blend ingredients and massage into affected areas.

Compress for Fevers

Materials

4-5 drops peppermint essential oil

Damp cloth

Directions

Apply peppermint essential oil to the damp cloth, squeezing to make sure that the oil mixes into the fabric. Apply compress to forehead for 15-20 minutes.

Fever Socks

Materials

4-5 drops tea tree oil
1 C cold water

Cotton socks
2 plastic shopping bags

Directions

Mix water and tea tree oil. Place socks in water, making sure that they are thoroughly soaked. Place socks on feet, and wrap with plastic shopping bags. Wear for 15-20 minutes at a time.

Sore Throat Gargle

Materials

½ C warm water
1-2 drops eucalyptus essential oil

1 tsp powdered ginger

Directions

Mix all ingredients and gargle to ease a sore throat.

Sinus Steam

Materials

8-10 drops peppermint essential oil
3-4 cups boiling water

Glass bowl
Towel

Directions

Place peppermint oil and boiling water in a glass bowl. Lean over the bowl, covering your head and the bowl with the towel. Inhale the vapors to clear your sinuses and ease congestion.

Essential Oil Cold Sore Treatment

Materials

8 drops geranium essential oil
3 drops lemon essential oil
8 drops tea tree oil

6 drops lavender essential oil
5 drops chamomile essential oil

Directions

Mix all ingredients together and store in a dark glass bottle. Apply one drop of mixture to a cotton ball or swat, and apply to the cold sore once daily.

Sinus-Ease Humidifier Blend

Materials

5 drops eucalyptus or peppermint
essential oil

Humidifier

Directions

Add essential oil to your humidifier. This will distribute the oil evenly throughout your home to make breathing easier.

Swollen Ankle Massage Oil

Materials

6 tsp evening primrose oil
15 drops fennel essential oil

15 drops Cyprus essential oil

Directions

Massage oil into legs, from the feet up to the knees to help alleviate ankle swelling. Remember to drink plenty of water as well.

How to Have Your Own Essential Oils Spa Party

If you are looking for a fun evening with your girlfriends, why not have a spa party? This is a great way to enjoy time with your friends, and have some refreshing facials, hand massages, and more. You can even go all out and have someone there to do makeup and manicures/pedicures. Hosting a spa party is easy, and you don't need to spend a lot of money, especially when you are making your own skin care products with essential oils.

Invitations

The first thing you need to do is choose a date for your essential oils spa party, and then do up/send out invitations. You can either create hand-written invitation and send them out via regular mail, or send them online through email or social networking sites. Be sure to include the date, time, and any special instructions, such as items to bring or clothing to wear.

Supplies and Decorations

Next, you will need to decorate for your essential oils spa party. You want to have a peaceful spa atmosphere, so loads of candles are a must, and scented candles are even better. Set up seating so there are tables with a variety of hand creams, face masks, and other spa items. Don't forget sweet treats, such as chocolates.

Set up stations for various services. For instance, if you are having facials, manicures/pedicures, hand massages, foot massages, etc., make sure that there is a separate station for each service. There should also be a relaxation area, where everyone can just sit and chat and enjoy a glass of wine.

Supplies and decorations you will need include, but are not limited to:
- Scented candles
- Candle holders
- Various treatments
- Manicure tools and polishes
- Makeup
- Hair styling items
- Cotton balls
- Cotton swabs
- Washcloths
- Bowls of water
- Foot soak basins
- Flowers

Food

You will need to feed your guests, but unlike other types of parties where pizzas, tacos, and other heavy foods are popular, you will want to serve light snacks. Some ideal suggestions include:

- Fresh fruit and veggie trays

- Cracker trays
- Dips
- Chocolates
- Cookies
- Cheese trays
- Deli platter
- Finger sandwiches
- Coffee and tea
- Wine
- Juice
- Water
- Petite fours
- Canapes

Activities

While there will be plenty going on with all of the various beauty treatments, you may still want to offer other activities for your guests, such as games with prizes. If you know that a lot of your guests aren't going to know each other, a great game idea is a conversation icebreaker where each person shares their name and an interesting piece of information about themselves. Trivia games are also popular, and winners can receive your home-made essential oil beauty treatments as prizes. If you can afford to have professional services, you may also want to have estheticians, makeup artists, manicurists, etc. do treatments on your guests.

Another idea for an activity is to have your guests make their own essential oil beauty treatments. You supply all of the ingredients, and they decide which items they wish to make. You can find loads of great recipes right here in this book that are ideal for essential oil spa parties. Make sure that you have plenty of pretty bottles and jars to hold the completed recipes (you can get these at your nearest dollar store).

Prizes

There are all kinds of options you can use for prizes to give to guests at your party. You may want to do up a big gift basket as a main prize, and fill it with various lotions, creams, soaps, etc. that you have made using essential oils. Don't forget to include accessories, such as bath puffs, sponges, and soft wash cloths.

February

February is the main month for romance, and we have plenty of romantic perfumes, aroma therapy treatments, spa treatments, massage oils, and more that will definitely put you in the mood for romance. Also, look for some delicious food treats and drinks, as well as more skin care and aroma therapy treatments for various types of issues and disorders.

VALENTINE'S DAY SCENT FOR WOMEN

Materials

6 drops bergamot essential oil
5 drops jasmine essential oil

6 drops sandalwood essential oil

Directions

Make perfumes according to the directions in the "How to Make Your Own Perfumes Using Essential Oils" in this book.

VALENTINE'S DAY SCENT FOR MEN

Materials

6 drops lime essential oil
8 drops sandalwood essential oil

5 drops coriander essential oil

Directions

Make perfumes according to the directions in the "How to Make Your Own Perfumes Using Essential Oils" in this book.

LUXURIOUS CLEANSER

Materials

½ C sweet almond oil
3 drops lavender essential oil
1 tbsp grated beeswax

1 tbsp pure distilled water
1 drop frankincense essential oil

Directions

In a double boiler over medium heat, combine beeswax and sweet almond oil. Place a Pyrex jar in a pan of simmering water, and add the distilled water. When the wax and oil are melted, add the warm distilled water, drop by drop. Remove from heat after adding half of the water. Add the rest of the water by drops, mixing with a whisk. Add the essential oils when the mixture begins to thicken. Pour into jars, cover, and label with the date.

EYE CREAM

Materials

2 tsp avocado oil
6 tsp carrot infused oil

½ C rosewater
1 tbsp grated beeswax

Directions

In a double boiler over medium heat, combine avocado oil, carrot infused oil, and beeswax. Add rosewater to a Pyrex jar, and place in a pan with simmering water. As the wax and oils melt together, begin adding the warm rosewater, drop by drop. When half of the rosewater has been added, remove from heat and slowly add the remaining rosewater, stirring with a whisk. When it thickens, pour into clean jars, cover, and label with the date.

SHAVING CREAM   February 5

Materials

4 tbsp coconut oil
2 tbsp avocado oil
1 C cocoa butter
3-4 tbsp witch hazel

4 drops carrot essential oil
8 drops lavender essential oil
1 tbsp cucumber juice (made from a fresh cucumber using a juicer or blender)

Directions

In a double boiler over medium heat, melt the cocoa butter. Remove from heat and add coconut oil and avocado oil, followed by the witch hazel. Add the cucumber juice and essential oils, and mix well. Pour mixture into clean glass jars. Cover and label with the date, and store in the refrigerator for up to two weeks.

NECK CREAM   February 6

Materials

½ C avocado oil
½ C wheat germ oil
2 tbsp grated beeswax
2 tbsp chamomile water

2 vitamin E capsules
8 drops chamomile essential oil
6 drops geranium essential oil
5 drops lemon essential oil

Directions

In a double boiler over medium heat, combine beeswax, wheat germ oil, and avocado oil. Add chamomile water to a Pyrex jar, and place in a pan with simmering water. When the wax and oils have melted and mixed, break open the vitamin E capsules, and add the liquid to this mixture. Next, add the chamomile water, drop by drop. When you have added half of the water, remove the mixture from heat and continue adding the rest of the water. As mixture thickens, add essential oils, stirring with a whisk. Pour mixture into clean jars. Cover, and label with the date.

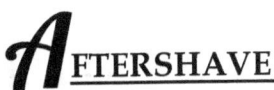

AFTERSHAVE

Materials

3 tbsp rubbing alcohol
2 tbsp witch hazel
2 tbsp pure distilled water
1-2 tbsp glycerin

10 drops cinnamon essential oil
25 drops orange essential oil
5 drops clove essential oil

Directions

Mix 1 tbsp alcohol with the essential oils, and blend well. In another jar, add the rest of the alcohol, distilled water, witch hazel, and glycerin, making sure the ingredients are well-mixed. Slowly add the essential oil and alcohol mixture to the second mixture, again making sure that all of the ingredients are mixed. Pour into dark glass bottles. Cover, and label with the date. Store in the fridge or another cool, dark place for up to two weeks.

ELBOW CREAM

Materials

½ C cocoa butter
½ C avocado oil
2 tbsp grated beeswax
2 vitamin E capsules

2 tbsp rosewater
8 drops lavender essential oil
6 drops orange essential oil

Directions

In a double boiler over medium heat, combine beeswax, avocado oil, and cocoa butter. Place rosewater in a Pyrex jar, and put into a pan of simmering water. When the wax and oils have melted and mixed together, break open the vitamin E capsules and add the liquid to the mixture. Add the rosewater drop by drop, until you have used half. Remove mixture from heat, and slowly add the rest of the rosewater, stirring with a whisk. As the mixture thickens, add the essential oils and continue to stir. Pour mixture into clean glass jars. Cover, and label with the date.

LUSCIOUS, KISSABLE LIP BALM

Materials

1 tsp raw honey
1 tsp cocoa butter
3 tbsp grated beeswax

4 tbsp rice bran oil
3 drops lavender essential oil
3 drops rose essential oil

Directions

In a double boiler over medium heat, combine beeswax, honey, cocoa butter, and rice bran oil. When ingredients have melted and mixed together, remove from heat and stir. As it cools down, add the essential oils. Pour mixture into lip balm tubs, cover, and label with the date.

Hot and Spicy Lip Balm

Materials

5 tbsp beeswax
3 tbsp rice bran oil

4-5 drops cinnamon essential oil
1 tbsp liquid aloe vera

Directions

In a double boiler over medium heat, combine beeswax, rice bran oil, and aloe vera. When wax melts and the ingredients have melted together, remove from heat and stir. When mixture thickens, add the cinnamon essential oil. Pour into lip balm tubes or tubs.

Chicken Alfredo

Materials

1 pound boneless, skinless chicken breast, cubed
½ C butter
1 C heavy cream
2 C shredded parmesan cheese (fresh)
1 clove garlic, crushed

Salt and pepper to taste
1 tbsp soya sauce
4 drops orange essential oil
5 drops basil essential oil
2 tbsp olive oil

Directions

Preheat oven to 350 degrees. In a frying pan, heat the olive oil. Add the chicken, followed by the soya sauce, essential oils, and some pepper. Cook until chicken is no longer pink inside. While chicken is cooking, combine shredded parmesan cheese, heavy cream, garlic, salt, and pepper in a food processor and blend until everything is well mixed. Transfer to a sauce pan, and heat over medium-low heat until cheese is completely melted. Place cooked chicken in a casserole dish, and cover with Alfredo sauce and more grated cheese. Bake for 20 minutes. Serve with your favorite pasta.

Baked Ham Glaze

Materials

1 C packed brown sugar
1 can pineapple slices in juice
4 drops wild orange essential oil
2 drops clove essential oil

½ C vinegar
½ C maple syrup (table syrup can be substituted)
1 tbsp mustard (honey mustard is a great substitution)

Directions

Combine brown sugar, essential oils, vinegar, maple syrup, mustard, and juice from pineapples (save pineapples to place on the ham while it is baking) in a saucepan, and heat over medium-low heat until sugar is completely dissolved. Remove from heat, and baste ham every half hour until cooked. In the last few minutes of baking, pour the remainder of the glaze over the ham, and cook uncovered so it gets good and sticky.

Puffy Eyes Blend

Materials

1 tbsp witch hazel
1 drop fennel essential oil

3 drops chamomile essential oil
2 tsp rice bran oil

Directions

Put the witch hazel in a glass bottle, and add the essential oils and rice bran oil. Keep this mixture in the refrigerator for the best results, and for a cooling relief for tired eyes. Apply by wrapping a piece of cotton around an ice cube, and dip this into the mixture. Place over your eyes and let it rest there for a few seconds.

Refreshing Body Scrub

Materials

1 C sugar
1/3 C coconut oil
3 tbsp orange zest

2 tbsp vegetable glycerin
8 drops peppermint essential oil
10 drops orange essential oil

Directions

Mix sugar, coconut oil, glycerin, and orange zest. You may need to use more or less oil to get the right consistency. Play around with it. Once this is mixed, slowly add the essential oils. Put sugar scrub into a glass container, label, and mark with the date.

Body Butter

Materials

1 ½ C solid coconut oil
3 tbsp raw honey
2 tbsp citrus zest

2-3 drops essential oil (same fruit as citrus zest)

Directions

Mix all ingredients until well blended and the mixture is nice and smooth. Pour into a container, cover, and label with the date.

Bath Melts

Materials

¼ C shea butter
¼ C cocoa butter
1 tsp lavender flowers

25 drops lavender essential oil
Silicone mold

Directions

In a double boiler over medium heat, melt the shea and coconut butters together. Add lavender flowers to mixture and stir. Remove from heat. Place a couple of drops of essential oil into each section of the silicone mold, and then add the butter mixture. Let everything cool, and then remove the bath melts from the mold and wrap to store.

Sweet-Smelling Pendant

Materials

Your favorite essential oil
Terra cotta clay
Clay stamps
Sand paper
Toothpick

Cutting mold (cookie cutter, bottle caps, etc.)
Scissors
Tin foil
Waxed paper

Directions

Rub some clay in your hands until it is easy to work with. Roll it out flat on top of the waxed paper until the clay is 1/8" thick. Use the cutting mold to create the pendant shape, and after removing excess clay, use the clay stamp to make a design on the pendant. Use the toothpick to create a hole for hanging the pendant from a chain or cord. You can also use any leftover clay to make smaller beads, using your toothpick to make the holes. Bake the pendant and beads according to the directions on the package of clay. Once the piece is cool, smooth it over with the sand paper, and then rub it with your favorite essential oil (one or two drops should do the trick nicely).

Lavender Bars

Materials

2 ounces beeswax
2 ounces coconut oil
2 ounces cocoa butter

15 drops lavender essential oil
1 tsp liquid aloe vera

Directions

In a double boiler over medium heat, combine beeswax, coconut oil, and shea butter. When they turn to liquid, remove from heat and add the essential oils, stirring to mix well. Pour mixture into silicone soap bar molds and let cool. Remove the bars from the molds and store in a cool, dry place. You can use extra beeswax if you want the bars to be firmer.

Copycat Burt's Bees Lip Balm   February 19

Materials

3 tbsp shaved beeswax
2 tbsp cocoa butter
¼ C sunflower oil
4 vitamin E capsules

2 drops rosemary essential oil
15 drops peppermint essential oil
Small drop of lanolin (no more than the size of a pea)

Directions

In a double boiler over medium heat, combine beeswax, cocoa butter, sunflower oil, and lanolin. Open the vitamin E capsules and add the liquid to the mixture. When the ingredients have melted together, remove from heat and add essential oils. Stir well with a whisk. When the mixture begins to cool, pour into lip balm tubes or tubs.

Body Wash   February 20

Materials

¼ C raw honey
¼ C coconut oil
½ C liquid Castile soap
3 vitamin E capsules

12 drops eucalyptus essential oil
15 drops sweet orange essential oil
10 drops lemon essential oil

Directions

Melt solid coconut oil in the microwave for 30 seconds or so until completely melted. Add raw honey, liquid from vitamin E capsules, and essential oils, stirring with a whisk. Next, add the Castile soap slowly, stirring, but gently so there are no bubbles. Pour mixture into bottles and shake before using.

Orange Body Spray   February 21

Materials

1 ounce pure distilled water
50-75 drops of orange essential (or whatever amount gives you the scent strength you prefer)

1 ounce witch hazel
½ tsp vegetable glycerine

Directions

Mix all ingredients well and pour into a spray bottle. Store in the refrigerator for a cool, refreshing spritz of scent. Remember to shake the ingredients well each time you use the body spray.

Patchouli Body Spray February 22

Materials

1 ounce pure distilled water
1 ounce witch hazel

½ tsp vegetable glycerine
1/8 tsp patchouli

Directions

Mix all ingredients well and pour into a spray bottle. Store in the refrigerator for a cool, refreshing spritz of scent. Remember to shake the ingredients well each time you use the body spray.

Home-Made Dish Soap February 23

Materials

¼ C unscented soap flakes
1 ½ C hot water

¼ C glycerin
5 drops lemon essential oil

Directions

In a double boiler over medium heat, melt the soap flakes and glycerin in the hot water. Remove from heat and let cool. When the mixture cools, add the lemon essential oil. Store in an old dish liquid squirt bottle.

All-Purpose Cleaner February 24

Materials

2 C water
2 tbsp mildly-scented dishwashing liquid
(lemon)

5 drops lemon essential oil

Directions

Combine all ingredients and put them into a spray bottle. Shake well before each use to make sure that all of the ingredients are well-blended.

Dryer Sheets February 25

Materials

Your favorite essential oils
Unscented foam cleaning sheets (look in
fabric section and buy by the yard)

Directions

Blend your favorite essential oils to get the scent you want. Cut foam sheets into dryer sheet-sized pieces. Put a couple of drops of essential oil mixture onto each sheet, squeezing to make sure that the scent gets all over the foam sheets. Some ideas for scents include lavender/vanilla, lavender/rosemary, lemon/chamomile, and lemon/orange. Have fun coming up with your own special scents.

Pet Shampoo   February 26

Materials

10 ounces pure distilled water
2 ounces liquid aloe vera
1 tbsp liquid Castile soap
2 drops peppermint essential oil

2 drops eucalyptus essential oil
2 drops lavender essential oil
2 drops rosemary essential oil

Directions

Mix all ingredients together and pour into a plastic squirt bottle. Shake well and then have fun trying to get your pet into the bathtub.

Rub for Swollen Feet   February 27

Materials

3 drops ginger essential oil
2 drops cypress essential oil

2 drops lavender essential oil
30 ml olive oil

Directions

Combine all ingredients and rub onto swollen feet. This is a great mixture for swollen feet caused by pregnancy. It can be used on any part of the body that is swollen and sore.

Bath Oil to Relieve Exhaustion   February 28

Materials

10 drops lavender essential oil
10 drops grapefruit essential oil

10 drops coriander essential oil
30 ml olive oil

Directions

Mix all ingredients together and shake well. Pour into a bottle, cover, and label with the date. For baths, use 6 drops of the mixture. For a foot bath, use 3-4 drops, and the same for a body rub.

DRY SHAMPOO

Materials

4 drops rosemary essential oil
4 drops tea tree oil

4 drops lavender essential oil
25 grams unscented talc

Directions

Place the talc in a blender, and add the essential oils, drop by drop, mixing on low speed. Place mixture into a container that can be tightly sealed. Use 1-2 teaspoons when you need to wash your hair but don't have time for a shower.

MAKE YOUR OWN FACIAL CLAY MASKS

You can spend a lot of money on facial clay masks, or you can make your own for pennies per treatment, using healthy ingredients that include essential oils. It only takes a couple of minutes to whip up a facial treatment, and you can use ingredients that you know are going to give you the results you are seeking. Many recipes are great for anyone who has oily skin, and there are also recipes for dry and combination skin.

Types of Clay

The type of clay you use for your facial masks is extremely important. For instance, if you are looking to cleanse, exfoliate, soothe, and tone your skin, French clays are optimal. Clays also come in a variety of colors, and each color has specific uses and healing properties for your skin. Clay colors include:

- **Green** – Helps to remove toxins and ease skin inflammation. Green clay is great for acne treatments.
- **White** – This is a soothing clay that is great for all types of skin. It is the gentlest, so it is ideal for sensitive skin.
- **Red** – If you have dry or sensitive skin, this is one of the best clays to use for your masks.
- **Pink** – This clay is great for toning and revitalizing your skin, and it is a good cleanser.

Other types of clay that are popular for facial masks include kaolin clay, Fuller's Earth, and bentonite clay.

Making Facial Clay Masks

There are a variety of recipes for clay masks, and the ones you use will depend on your particular skin care needs. A basic clay mask recipe includes clay powder, distilled water or liquid aloe vera, essential oils, and vitamin E from vitamin capsules. The masks are applied as any other facial mask. Allow the mask to dry for 20 minutes to a half an hour, and remove with lukewarm water.

March

Spring is just around the corner now, and it is time to start thinking about spring cleaning, new outfits, and of course, fresh scents. This month, you will find loads of recipes for delicious foods, pet care, body scrubs, lip balms, and a whole lot more. There are also plenty of recipes for baby products, including a formula for soothing diaper rash.

ℰgyptian Goddess Perfume

Materials

2 drops cinnamon essential oil
2 drops lime essential oil

5 drops rose essential oil
5 drops Ylang Ylang essential oil

Directions

Follow the directions in the section, "How to Make Your Own Perfumes Using essential Oils".

Cleansing Body Scrub

Materials

1 tbsp oat bran
2 tbsp extra virgin olive oil

1 tbsp wheat germ
3 drops orange essential oil

Directions

Combine oat bran and wheat germ. Add almond oil, and stir to create a paste. Blend in the orange essential oil. Use this scrub sparingly, and it will cover all of your skin. Rinse with warm water.

Facial Toner

Materials

½ C pure distilled water
½ C rosewater
2 drops chamomile essential oil

4 drops lavender essential oil
2 drops geranium essential oil

Directions

Combine distilled water and rosewater in a dark glass bottle. Add the essential oils, and shake. Cover, and label with the date. Storing the mixture in the refrigerator will not only give it a longer life, it will feel even more refreshing when you use it.

Cleansing Mask

Materials

1 ounce green clay
3 tbsp pure distilled water
1 tsp vegetable glycerin

3 drops grapefruit essential oil
1 drop juniper essential oil

Directions

Follow the instructions that are provided in the "How to Make Clay Facial Masks with Essential Oils" section of this book.

Refreshing Foot Bath

Materials

2 drops lemongrass essential oil
4 drops lime essential oil

3 drops geranium essential oil

Directions

Fill a basin with warm water. Add the essential oils, and stir to make sure that they are well distributed throughout the water. Use this foot soak for up to 15 minutes or until the water starts to cool off.

Acne Treatment

March 6

Materials

3 tbsp jojoba oil
6 drops lavender essential oil

4 drops tea tree oil essential
2 drops geranium essential oil

Directions

Combine all of the ingredients in a dark glass bottle. Shake well. Store in the refrigerator for a longer life. Apply to any area of the skin where acne is an issue, twice daily.

Hand Treatment

March 7

Materials

2 tbsp extra virgin olive oil
1 tsp raw honey
2 tbsp jojoba oil

1 tbsp rosewater
8 drops lemon essential oil

Directions

In a double boiler over medium heat, combine honey, olive oil, and jojoba oil and melt the ingredients together. Heat rosewater in a second double boiler. When the oils have melted together and the rosewater is warm, add the rosewater drop by drop. When half of the rosewater has been added, remove from heat and continue to slowly add the rest of the rosewater. Stir with a whisk, and then add the lemon essential oil. Pour into a jar, cover, and label with the date.

Face Gel Acne Blend

March 8

Materials

4 tbsp aloe vera gel
2 drops juniper essential oil

4 drops lavender essential oil
4 drops tea tree oil

Directions

Combine aloe vera gel and essential oils in a jar. Stir well with a cosmetic spatula to completely blend the ingredients. Cover and label with the date. To use, apply a small amount to your face and neck and gently massage the skin. Rinse with warm water and pat skin dry.

Face Gel Dry Skin Blend   March 9

Materials

4 tbsp aloe vera gel
4 drops carrot essential oil

2 drops chamomile essential oil
3 drops sandalwood essential oil

Directions

Combine aloe vera gel and essential oils in a jar. Stir well with a cosmetic spatula to completely blend the ingredients. Cover and label with the date. To use, apply a small amount to your face and neck and gently massage the skin. Rinse with warm water and pat skin dry.

Face Gel Problem Skin Blend   March 10

Materials

4 tbsp aloe vera gel
4 drops carrot essential oil

3 drops geranium essential oil
3 drops parsley essential oil

Directions

Combine aloe vera gel and essential oils in a jar. Stir well with a cosmetic spatula to completely blend the ingredients. Cover and label with the date. To use, apply a small amount to your face and neck and gently massage the skin. Rinse with warm water and pat skin dry.

Shower Gel   March 11

Materials

1 C shower gel base
10 drops orange essential oil
10 drops lemon essential oil

5 drops grapefruit essential oil
1 tbsp aloe vera gel

Directions

Put the shower gel base in a pump bottle. Add each essential oil separately, shaking after adding each oil. Label with the date and store in a cool, dark place.

Puffy Eye Tonic

Materials

1 C rosewater
1 tsp castor oil

1 drop rose essential oil
2 tbsp cornflower petals

Directions

Chop up the cornflower petals and put in a saucepan with rosewater. Simmer for 15-20 minutes. Let cool, and pour into a jar. Add the castor oil and rose essential oil, and shake well. Cover and abel with the date. Store in the fridge. To use, soak cotton balls or pads in the solution, and place on your eyes for 10 minutes or longer.

All Over Moisturizer

Materials

1 tbsp aloe vera gel
1 tbsp carrot-infused oil
5 drops lavender essential oil

6 drops geranium essential oil
2 drops rose essential oil
3 tbsp sweet almond oil

Directions

Combine all ingredients into a ceramic bowl, and beat with an electric mixer until the mixture begins to thicken. Pour into a glass jar, cover, and label with the date. The ingredients may separate as the mixture sits, so be sure to shake it before each use.

Anti-Aging Mask

Materials

½ C pure distilled water
1 tbsp red clay
1 ounce slippery elm powder

2 drops bergamot essential oil
2 drops chamomile essential oil
1 drop immortelle essential oil

Directions

Combine distilled water and slippery elm powder in a saucepan and simmer for 20-25 minutes. Remove from heat, strain, and let cool. Add clay and blend. Add the essential oils, and blend again with a spoon. Apply all over damp facial and neck skin, and let sit for 20 minutes.

Rose Moisturizer

Materials

3 tbsp extra virgin olive oil
1 tbsp rosehip oil
1 tsp avocado oil
3 tbsp rosewater

½ C glycerin
8 drops rose essential oil
5 drops rosewood essential oil
1 drop lavender essential oil

Directions

Combine all ingredients in a ceramic or glass bowl, and mix with an electric mixer until mixture begins to thicken. Pour into a glass jar, cover, and label with the date.

Relaxation Perfume

Materials

4 drops cedarwood essential oil
2 drops clary sage essential oil

1 drop grapefruit essential oil
2 drops mandarin orange essential oil

Directions

Follow the directions in the section, "How to Make Your Own Perfumes Using essential Oils".

Fruit Salsa

Materials

5-6 C chopped fruit
3 tbsp orange preserves

2 drops tangerine essential oil
1 drop citrus blend essential oil

Directions

Combine all of the ingredients in a large bowl. Place in the refrigerator to chill for one half hour before serving.

Cinnamon Chips

Materials

4 tbsp agave
3 drops cinnamon bark essential oil

4 tortillas, cut into triangles
Raw coconut oil

Directions

Preheat oven to 350 degrees. Mix cinnamon essential oil and agave. Brush one side of tortilla wedges with coconut oil, and brush the other side with the cinnamon oil mixture. Lay out flat on a cookie sheet, and cook for 8-10 minutes or until slightly brown and crispy. Let cool and serve with fruit salsa.

Garden Smoothie

Materials

1 beet (medium-sized)
1 cucumber
1 small bunch grapes (about the size of a handful)

2 Swiss chard leaves
2 kale leaves
1 drop fennel essential oil
1 C filtered water

Directions

Combine all ingredients in a blender and mix until smooth.

Anti-Wrinkle Oil

Materials

10 drops lavender essential oil
10 drops fennel essential oil
2 drops rosemary essential oil
10 drops neroli essential oil
10 drops frankincense essential oil

10 drops evening primrose essential oil
10 drops carrot essential oil
3 drops lemon essential oil
2 tbsp apricot kernel oil

Directions

Mix all of the essential oils into the apricot kernel oil. Apply to the skin on the face and neck every night, massaging into the skin.

Pine Floor Cleaner

Materials

6 drops pine essential oil
3 drops cypress essential oil

1 gallon warm water

Directions

Stir essential oils into the warm water. Use on floors immediately.

Carpet Deodorizer

Materials

1 C baking soda
6 drops sweet orange essential oil
3 drops cinnamon essential oil

Directions

Combine all baking soda and essential oils, mixing well. Sprinkle onto carpet. Allow mixture to sit on carpet for 5-10 minutes, and then vacuum as normal.

CITRUS DISHWASHING LIQUID   March 23

Materials

20 ounces liquid castile soap
20 drops lime essential oil

10 drops sweet orange essential oil
5 drops citrus seed extract

Directions

Combine castile soap, essential oils, and citrus seed extract into a squeeze bottle. Shake before each use. When using, add 1-2 tablespoons to dishwater and agitate to get the water sudsy.

OVEN CLEANER   March 24

Materials

¼ C washing soda
1 box baking soda
½ C table salt
¼ C water

¾ C vinegar
10 drops lemon essential oil
10 drops thyme essential oil

Directions

In a glass bowl, combine washing soda, baking soda, and salt. Add enough water to create a paste. Spread this paste on the oven racks and walls, and let sit for 20-30 minutes (oven pre-heated to 250 degrees). Mix vinegar and essential oils in a spray bottle. Spray the oven walls and racks with this mixture, then wipe clean with a damp cloth and rinse well.

FLEA REPELLANT   March 25

Materials

10 drops peppermint essential oil

2 ounces mild organic soap

Directions

Mix ingredients and apply to pets' skin and fur with a spray bottle. This needs to be done a few times daily, as this mixture is not as strong as commercially-prepared flea repellants. The upside is that it is also not as harsh and dangerous to your pets.

Stretch Mark Formula

Materials

30 ml extra virgin olive oil
15 ml wheat germ oil

10 drops borage seed essential oil
5 drops carrot essential oil

Directions

Combine ingredients in a glass bottle. Cover and label with the date. Shake well before each use. Apply to area where you have stretch marks.

Alopecia Shampoo

Materials

100 ml shampoo base
15 drops jojoba oil
8 drops carrot essential oil

7 drops rosemary essential oil
7 drops lavender essential oil
2 drops tea tree oil

Directions

Combine all ingredients in a squeeze or pump bottle. Use instead of your regular shampoo for alopecia.

Hair Loss Lotion

Materials

50 ml rosewater
50 ml pure distilled water
5 drops rosemary essential oil

6 drops jojoba oil
3 drops carrot essential oil
3 drops geranium essential oil

Directions

Combine all ingredients in a glass jar. Cover, label with the date, and store in the refrigerator. Shake before each use. To use, apply two teaspoons of mixture and massage into scalp.

Diaper Rash Treatment

Materials

1 pint warm water
1 drop German chamomile essential oil

1 drop lavender essential oil

Directions

Combine ingredients and store in a glass jar. Apply by dipping a cotton ball into the liquid and wipe the affected area.

COUGH SOLUTION FOR BABIES AND CHILDREN March 30

Materials

3 drops eucalyptus essential oil or eucalyptus smithi

Vaporizer

Directions

Add eucalyptus essential oil to the vaporizer. The steam will release the healing molecules in the essential oil into the room. This should not be used on babies younger than two months.

POISE PERFUME March 31

Materials

2 drops basil essential oil
3 drops bergamot essential oil

1 drop coriander essential oil
4 drops petit grain essential oil

Directions

Follow the directions in the section, "How to Make Your Own Perfumes Using essential Oils".

How to Make Your Own Perfumes Using Essential Oils

Often, you are on the search for the perfect scent, only to find that what you really want doesn't even exist. There may be scents out there that are close to what you want, but they are missing something. You know, it is super-easy to make your own perfumes, and you don't need to have a chemist's lab set up in your home. All you need are a few tools that you probably already have, and some ingredients which you can order from any company that carries essential oils and supplies. Let's get started.

Perfume Base

The first thing you will need is a good base for your perfume. Some people recommend alcohol, while others recommend a carrier oil. The ideal solution will be a blend of carrier oil and alcohol. Vodka is the best choice, as it is pretty much odorless. For a carrier oil, jojoba is the best, although also the most expensive. While you are learning to make your own perfume, it may be better to use a cheaper carrier oil, such as apricot kernel oil. Once you get the scent right, you can switch it up and use the higher-quality jojoba oil.

Necessary Equipment

Once you have chosen the ingredients for your perfume base, you will need to gather up all of the equipment you need to make perfume. You will need measuring spoons, a small funnel, and a small bottle to store your perfume (colored bottles are best because they don't let a lot of light in that will diminish the scent over time).

Making Perfume at Home

Mix equal amounts of carrier oil and alcohol (about a teaspoon each) into the glass bottle. Add your favorite essential oils, one drop at a time, shaking well after the addition of each drop. Cover the bottle and store for at least two weeks. Shake mixture three times a day during the storage period. Experiment with various essential oils to come up with your own signature scent.

April

Now that spring is finally here, it is time to really get into the spring cleaning, even more than last month. We have all kinds of great recipes for cleaning products for your home, as well as many other recipes for perfumes, skin care, hair care, and lots more. Read on.

Cough Drops

Materials

1 C raw honey
1 tsp butter
8 drops Thieves essential oil

7 drops lemon essential oil
2 drops eucalyptus essential oil

Directions

In a sauce pan over medium-low heat, combine the butter and raw honey. Stir frequently, and turn heat down after mixture comes to a boil. Cook for about 20 minutes, or until a candy thermometer reads 300 degrees. Remove from heat, and add essential oils as the mixture cools and thickens. Drop by teaspoons onto a cookie sheet lined with parchment paper and allow to cool. Placed cooled lozenges in an airtight container.

Lemongrass Scrub

Materials

4 tbsp sugar
2 tsp sweet almond oil
3 drops geranium essential oil

3 drops fennel essential oil
12 drops lemongrass essential oil

Directions

Combine ingredients together in a jar. Cover and label with the date. This mixture is best when used after you have taken a bath or a shower and your skin is warm and moist.

Sensitive Skin Clay Mask

Materials

2 ounces red clay
6 tbsp rosewater
2 tsp jojoba oil

5 drops chamomile essential oil
3 drops rose essential oil

Directions

Follow the directions in the "Make Your Own Facial Clay Masks" section in this book.

Exfoliating Body Scrub

Materials

¼ C coarse sea salt
¼ C Epsom salts

¼ C grapeseed oil
2 drops lavender essential oil

Directions

Put the salt into a Mason jar, and cover with grapeseed oil. Add the essential oils and stir to mix everything together. Apply this scrub to damp skin, massaging it into the skin using circular motions. Do not use this mixture on skin that has cuts or scratches, because it will sting. Rinse with warm water and pat dry.

Doggie Flea Collar 1   April 5

Materials

Fabric dog collar to fit your dog comfortably

2 tbsp almond oil
2-3 drops peppermint essential oil

Directions

Combine the almond oil and peppermint essential oil in a bowl. Place the collar in the bowl, and make sure that it is completely soaked in the solution and allow to dry. You will need to re-do the flea solution on the collar every couple of weeks. This can also be used for cats, but only use one drop of peppermint essential oil as their skin is sensitive.

Doggie Flea Collar 2   April 6

Materials

Bandana or other fabric that will comfortably fit around your dog's neck

10 drops citronella essential oil
10 drops eucalyptus essential oil

Directions

Lay the fabric out flat and cover it with the essential oils by placing drops all over the fabric. Allow to dry. Remember to replenish the flea solution every two weeks or so.

Heartburn Relief   April 7

Materials

1 tbsp raw honey
1 drop coriander essential oil

1 drop cardamom essential oil
1 drop dill essential oil

Directions

Combine honey and essential oils in a dark glass bottle. Shake to blend all of the ingredients together. Store in a cool dark place. To use, add half of the mixture to some warm soya milk and enjoy twice a day after meals.

Baby Massage Oil

Materials

2 tbsp sweet almond oil

1-2 drops lavender essential oil

Directions

Mix sweet almond oil and lavender essential oil, and give your baby a nice, relaxing massage. After the age of two months, you can increase the amount of essential oil to four or five drops.

Foamy Carpet Shampoo

Materials

6 C water
1 ½ C liquid castile soap

20 drops peppermint essential oil

Directions

Combine all of the ingredients together in a blender until mixture is foamy. Rub the foam into dirty areas of your carpet with a sponge. Allow to dry, and then vacuum as normal to get rid of the dirt and any remaining foam.

Toilet Bowl Cleaner

Materials

2 C water
¼ C liquid castile soap

1 tbsp tea tree oil
10 drops peppermint essential oil

Directions

Add all of the ingredients to a spray bottle. Shake well to mix the ingredients together. Spray on the inside of the toilet bowl, and on all of the surfaces to disinfect the whole toilet. Wipe with a damp cloth.

Toothpaste

Materials

6 tbsp bentonite clay
4 tbsp coconut oil, liquefied
2 tsp ground green stevia
1 ½ tsp high mineral salt
2 tsp baking soda

3 tbsp pure distilled water, or more if needed
¼ tsp peppermint essential oil
¼ tsp Thieves oil

Directions

Blend stevia, coconut oil, baking soda, salt, and essential oil in a glass bowl. Stir until mixture is thoroughly blended. Add the clay, and then begin to add the water slowly. When the mixture reaches the consistency of toothpaste, it is ready to use. Put it into a pump bottle instead of worrying about making a mess trying to get the toothpaste into a tube.

GARLIC AND HERB CHICKEN   April 12

Materials

1 small chicken
4 cloves fresh garlic, finely minced
½ drop thyme essential oil
½ drop rosemary essential oil
1 medium onion, finely minced

½ tsp poultry seasoning
2 tsp salt
1 tsp ground black pepper
1 ½ tsp olive oil

Directions

Preheat oven to 325 degrees. Combine all of the oils and herbs together in a glass bowl. Rub the mixture all over the chicken, making sure to get it under the skin and inside the cavity. Place chicken in a roaster, brush with olive oil, and bake until juices run clear when meat is pierced (about 2 hours or so).

CILANTRO SALAD DRESSING   April 13

Materials

1 C Miracle Whip salad dressing
1 drop cilantro essential oil
½ tsp cayenne pepper

2 cloves garlic, minced
1 tsp paprika
1 package Ranch dressing mix

Directions

Combine all of the ingredients in a blender. Pour into a jar and refrigerate for a couple of hours before serving. You can make this dressing thicker by using less mayo and adding some sour cream.

YOGURT DIP   April 14

Materials

1 tub plain Greek yogurt
1 tbsp raw honey

4-5 drops wild orange essential oil

Directions

Mix all of the ingredients together in a glass bowl. Cover, and refrigerate for a couple of hours before serving. Serve with a variety of fresh fruits.

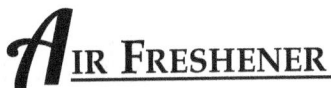IR FRESHENER

Materials

25 drops peppermint essential oil
5 drops lemon essential oil

1 ounce of pure distilled water

Directions

Combine all of the ingredients into a spray bottle. Shake well to blend all of the ingredients. To use, spray in any area of your house where you want a lemony/minty fresh scent.

CITRUS MINT DIFFUSER BLEND April 16

Materials

6 drops grapefruit essential oil
1 drop lemon essential oil

3 drops spearming essential oil

Directions

Follow the directions in the "Using Aromatherapy Diffusers" section in this book.

SLEEPY TIME PILLOW SPRAY April 17

Materials

15 ml pure distilled water
2 drops lavender essential oil
2 drops chamomile essential oil

1 drop sweet orange essential oil
1 drop Ylang Ylang essential oil

Directions

Combine all ingredients into a spray bottle. Shake well to thoroughly mix the ingredients. Spray on pillow cases and let dry.

BACKACHE MASSAGE OIL 1 April 18

Materials

2 tbsp extra virgin olive oil
10 drops lavender essential oil
5 drops sandalwood essential oil

5 drops rosemary essential oil
3 drops geranium essential oil

Directions

Combine all of the ingredients in a dark glass bottle (amber is the best choice because it doesn't let light in). Shake well to thoroughly blend all of the ingredients. Apply and massage into affected areas.

*B*ACKACHE MASSAGE OIL 2

Materials

1 C sweet almond oil
12 drops black pepper essential oil
6 drops juniper berry essential oil

5 drops ginger essential oil
5 drops marjoram essential oil

Directions

Combine all of the ingredients in a dark glass bottle (amber is the best choice because it doesn't let light in). Shake well to thoroughly blend all of the ingredients. Apply and massage into affected areas. This can be used for all of your aching muscles, and not just your back.

*B*UBBLE GUM/MINT LIP BALM

Materials

3 tbsp shredded beeswax
1 tbsp cocoa butter
1 tsp sweet almond oil

1 vitamin E capsule
2 drops peppermint essential oil
2 drops bubblegum lip balm flavor

Directions

In a double boiler over medium heat, combine beeswax, coconut butter, and sweet almond oil. When the wax has melted and the ingredients have blended together, remove from heat and add the liquid from the vitamin E capsule, peppermint essential oil, and bubblegum flavor. Pour mixture into lip balm tubes or tubs and allow to set for a few hours before using.

*G*EL AIR FRESHENER

Materials

2 envelopes unflavored gelatin
½ C boiling water
½ C ice water

12 drops apple essential oil
5-6 drops red food coloring
1 tbsp salt

Directions

Dissolve the gelatin in the boiling water. Add the ice water, followed by the apple essential oil and salt. If you want to make it colorful, add the food coloring. Pour mixture into small jars, cover, and let cool overnight. To use, simply open a jar and place it on a warm stovetop, on a shelf, or even inside your vehicle in a cup holder.

$\mathcal{D}$ETOXIFYING HAIR MASK

Materials

½ C bentonite clay powder
½ C aloe vera gel

1 ¼ C apple cider vinegar
5 drops rosemary essential oil

Directions

Mix clay, essential oil, aloe vera gel, and ¼ cup of the apple cider vinegar and massage through hair. Cover with a shower cap or plastic wrap, and let it sit on the hair for about one half hour, but be sure not to let it dry. Rinse hair with the rest of the vinegar, and sit for about three minutes before shampooing as usual.

$\mathcal{P}$IMPLE RELIEF

Materials

2 tbsp coconut oil
3-4 drops Purification Oil blend

Lip balm tubes

Directions

In a double boiler over medium heat, melt the coconut oil. Remove from heat and add the essential oil, stirring to mix well. Use a dropper to pour the mixture into lip balm tubes. Let sit for an hour or so to set, and store in the refrigerator to keep it from melting. To use, apply to pimples when you see them.

$\mathcal{I}$NSECT REPELLENT

Materials

2 tbsp witch hazel
2 tbsp grapeseed oil
½ tsp vodka (acts as a preservative)
55 drops lemon eucalyptus essential oil

20 drops cedarwood essential oil
20 drops lavender essential oil
20 drops rosemary essential oil

Directions

Combine witch hazel, grapeseed oil, and vodka in a spray bottle and shake well. Add the essential oils and shake again. Remember to shake every time you use to make sure that the ingredients are always well blended. Apply to the skin every couple of hours to keep bugs away.

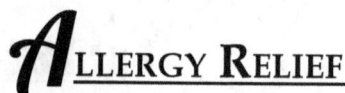 LLERGY RELIEF

Materials

Peppermint essential oil
Small bottle to wear as jewelry

Directions

Fill the bottle with essential oil, cap, and hang on a chain or silk/leather cord. Any time you feel an allergy sinus attack coming on, open the bottle and take a whiff. You can also apply a drop of peppermint essential oil at the base of your neck twice daily, or near your nostrils.

Diaper Rash Relief

Materials

3 tbsp grated beeswax
1 tbsp shea butter
2 tbsp coconut oil

1 tbsp jojoba oil
10 drops lavender essential oil
10 drops tea tree oil

Directions

In a double boiler over medium heat, combine beeswax, shea butter, jojoba oil, and coconut oil. When ingredients have melted and blended together, remove from heat and add the essential oils. Pour mixture to a deodorant container and let cool. Apply to diaper rash as needed.

Washing Machine Freshener

Materials

White vinegar

Lemon essential oil

Directions

Fill washing machine as normal with laundry, and add laundry detergent. Fill the bleach dispenser with vinegar, and add a couple of drops of lemon essential oil. Not only will this keep your washing machine smelling fresh, it will also soften the laundry and add a nice scent to your clothing.

Canker Sore Treatment

April 28

Materials

Thieves Oil
Coconut oil

Directions

Mix one drop of Thieves Oil in one tsp of coconut oil. Apply to the affected area, and repeat two to three times daily until the canker sore is gone.

Sweet-Smelling Wax Melts

April 29

Materials

2 ounces grated beeswax
2 tbsp coconut oil
10 drops Lavender essential oil

10 drops sweet orange essential oil
1 tbsp vanilla extract

Directions

In a double boiler over medium heat, combine beeswax and coconut oil. When they have melted together, remove from heat and stir in essential oils and vanilla extract. Pour into silicon wafer molds and let cool. To use, add as many as you want to a warmer and enjoy the sweet scent.

Ear Infection Remedy

April 30

Materials

5 ml grapeseed oil

1 drop clove essential oil

Directions

Mix ingredients, and massage around the ears and neck area for relief from earache infections.

HOUSE CLEANING WITH ESSENTIAL OILS

You want to have a clean, fresh-smelling home, but do you really want to use harsh chemical cleansers that are harmful to the environment, and can also be harmful to the health of you and your family? You know, you can save a lot of money, and have healthy cleansers for your home. All you have to do is make your own, using many ingredients that you already have, and a few essential oils. The home-made cleaners work just as well, if not better than the commercial cleaning products, and you can be sure that there are no dangerous chemicals in the products you use around your home.

Use Undiluted Essential Oils

It is important to always use essential oils that are pure and undiluted when you are making household cleaning solutions. Don't worry about the various grade differences, as this only refers to the actual scent and not the quality of the oils. Make sure that your essential oils are always stored in dark bottles (blue or brown is best so light can't get in and ruin the chemical properties of the oils), and store them in a cool place that is not in direct light. Most essential oils will remain potent for many years, with the exception of citrus oils, which are only good for a year or so.

Follow the Recipes to the Letter

If a recipe calls for a specific amount of an essential oil, it is imperative that you use that exact amount. This is because the oils are already highly concentrated, and using more isn't going to make much of a difference so you are just going to be wasting it. Because many essential oils can be hard on skin (tea tree oil is a good example of this), always wear rubber gloves when making your cleaning solutions, and keep these solutions away from small children and pets.

May

Summer is just around the corner, and it is time to start dusting off those lightweight summer clothes and opening the house to let the fresh air and sunshine in. You can make your whole home smell fresh and clean, and you don't even have to use commercial cleaning products. This month, we have all kinds of great recipes for home-made cleaning products. Of course, there are other awesome recipes as well, including delicious meals, hair and skin care, pet care, and a whole lot more.

SELF-CONFIDENCE PERFUME

Materials

4 drops rosemary essential oil
1 drop ginger essential oil

2 drops myrtle essential oil
3 drops verbena essential oil

Directions

Follow the directions in the "How to Make Your Own Perfumes Using Essential Oils" in this book.

BODY SCRUB

Materials

2 tbsp oatmeal (coarsely ground)
2 tbsp plain yogurt

4 drops lemon essential oil
15 ivy leaves

Directions

Combine ivy leaves, oatmeal, and yogurt until the consistency is smooth. Add lemon essential oil, and stir until mixture turns into a paste that is nice and smooth.

SKIN REVITALIZING MASK

Materials

2 ounces pink clay
6 tbsp orange flower water
2 tsp glycerin

2 drops neroli essential oil
4 drops orange essential oil
4 drops petit grain essential oil

Follow the directions in the "Make Your Own Facial Clay Masks" section of this book.

WRINKLE CREAM

Materials

1 tbsp grated beeswax
¼ C jojoba oil
¼ C rice bran oil
2 vitamin E capsules

1 tbsp rosewater
3 drops carrot essential oil
5 drops rosemary essential oil
3 drops fennel essential oil

Directions

In a double boiler over medium heat, combine beeswax, jojoba oil, and rice bran oil. In another double boiler over medium heat, add the rosewater. When the ingredients have melted and blended together, add the liquid from the vitamin E capsules and stir. Add half of the rosewater, drop by drop, to this mixture. Remove from heat, and add the rest of the water, stirring with a whisk. As the mixture thickens, add the essential oils. Pour mixture into glass jars, cover, and label with the date.

Hand Cream for Mom

Materials

4 tbsp grated beeswax
10 tbsp cocoa butter
4 tbsp rice bran oil
6 tbsp apricot oil

2 tbsp rosehip oil
15 drops geranium essential oil
12 drops Melissa essential oil
10 drops parsley essential oil

Directions

In a double boiler over medium heat, combine cocoa butter, rice bran oil, apricot oil, and rosehip oil, stirring constantly. When ingredients melt and blend together, remove from heat and continue stirring for another minute or so. Before the mixture thickens, add the essential oils, and stir again for another minute. Pour mixture into jars, cover, and label with the date. Allow to sit overnight before using. For best results, use twice daily.

Concentration Diffusion Blend

Materials

2 drops black pepper essential oil
2 drops coriander essential oil

2 drops geranium essential oil

Directions

Follow the directions in the "Using Aroma Therapy Diffusers" section of this book.

Pick-Me-Up Diffusion Blend

Materials

1 drop dill essential oil
2 drops bergamot essential oil

3 drops rosemary essential oil
2 drops coriander essential oil

Directions

Follow the directions in the "Using Aroma Therapy Diffusers" section of this book.

Kitchen Aroma Therapy

Materials

2 drops rosemary essential oil
3 drops lemon essential oil

1 drop basil essential oil

Directions

Follow the directions in the "Using Aroma Therapy Diffusers" section of this book.

Revitalizing Bath Oil

May 9

Materials

½ C rice bran oil
5 drops peppermint essential oil

1 drop pine essential oil
4 drops rosemary essential oil

Directions

Combine all of the ingredients in a glass bowl, and add to your bathwater. To make this bath even more revitalizing, add a bit of cold water at the end of your bath, or stand under a cool shower. Massage any remaining oil into your skin after you dry off.

Bath Fizzies

May 10

Materials

1 C bicarbonate of soda (baking soda)
½ C citric acid

10 drops lemon essential oil
10 drops orange essential oil

Directions

Mix the citric acid and soda together in a glass bowl, mixing well enough to remove all lumps. Next, add the essential oils, and blend thoroughly. Pack mixture into molds or even small muffin tins, and let sit overnight to harden. Use one or two in your bath.

Air Spray

May 11

Materials

2 C pure distilled water
5 drops cinnamon essential oil
5 drops Thyme essential oil
10 drops Bergamot essential oil
10 drops Citronella essential oil

5 drops Lemon essential oil
5 drops Sage essential oil
10 drops Lavender essential oil
5 drops Eucalyptus essential oil
10 drops Tea Tree essential oil

Directions

Combine all ingredients in a spray bottle. Shake well before using. This is a great spray to keep your bathroom smelling nice and fresh.

Easy Liquid Soap

May 12

Materials

2 C unscented liquid soap
5 drops lemon essential oil

10 drops sweet orange essential oil
5 drops grapefruit essential oil

365 Days of Essential Oils   55

Directions

Combine all ingredients in a soap pump bottle and shake gently to make sure everything is well blended without making it foamy.

Refreshing Body Oil

Materials

1 C rice bran oil
20 drops lemon grass essential oil

20 drops juniper essential oil
22 drops fennel essential oil

Directions

Combine all of the ingredients in a pump bottle. To use, apply to skin after showering or bathing, massing it into the areas where you have cellulite. This is a great detox mixture, and has a great scent that will wake you up.

Kitchen Cleaner

Materials

Water
20 drops lemon essential oil

10 drops sweet orange essential oil

Directions

Fill a dark glass bottle with water. Add the essential oils and shake well. To use, pour a bit of the mixture onto a cloth or a sponge and wipe down the area that needs to be cleaned.

Handbag Freshener

Materials

3 drops geranium essential oil
2 drops Melissa essential oil

3 drops bergamot essential oil

Directions

Apply the essential oils to a cotton ball, and place in your purse. Replace the cotton ball once a week to keep your purse smelling nice and fresh.

Man Bag Freshener

Materials

3 drops black pepper essential oil
1 drop clove essential oil

3 drops orange essential oil

Directions

Follow the directions as per the Hand Bag Freshener from above recipe.

Drawer Freshener

Materials

5 drops lavender essential oil

5 drops rosemary essential oil

Directions

Apply the essential oils to cotton balls or into a pomander. Place in drawers to keep them smelling fresh.

Kitchen Soap

Materials

1 C unscented liquid soap
3 drops lemon essential oil

6 drops coffee essential oil

Directions

In a glass bowl, combine liquid soap and essential oils, stirring gently to mix without creating bubbles. Pour into a pump bottle.

Jet Lag Swollen Ankle Formula

Materials

5 drops geranium essential oil

1 tbsp extra virgin olive oil

Directions

If your ankles swell when you are flying, blend these ingredients together and massage them into the skin on your ankles, feet, and calves before each flight.

Travel Sickness Blend

Materials

3 drops peppermint essential oil

1 tbsp extra virgin olive oil

Directions

Mix ingredients, and apply them to a handkerchief. Take a whiff periodically to avoid travel sickness. You can also rub this mixture onto your stomach to combat nausea.

INSECT REPELLENT

Materials

1 tbsp extra virgin olive oil or vegetable oil
6 drops citronella essential oil
10 drops lavender essential oil

8 drops peppermint essential oil
8 drops thyme essential oil

Directions

Combine all of the ingredients and massage into exposed areas of skin before going outside.

YLANG YLANG HAIR OIL

Materials

½ ounce jojoba oil
2 drops lavender essential oil

2 drops rose geranium essential oil
2 drops ylang ylang essential oil

Directions

Combine ingredients in an amber or other dark colored bottle. To use, massage into scalp, let sit for a couple of minutes, and then rinse, and shampoo as normal.

CUTICLE SOAK

Materials

1 tbsp liquid castile soap
3 drops lemon essential oil

3 drops lavender essential oil
3 drops sandalwood essential oil

Directions

Combine ingredients in a glass bowl, and stir gently to mix. Soak fingertips in this mixture for 5-10 minutes. This will soften your cuticles and make your nails nice and clean. If you have a problem with nail fungus, you can also add 3-4 drops of tea tree oil to the mixture.

ESSENTIAL OIL CANDIES

Materials

2 egg whites
4-5 C powdered sugar
Red food coloring

Cinnamon essential oil (or whatever flavor you prefer for your candies)

Directions

Beat egg whites until they are foamy but have not stiffened. Add some of the powdered sugar, and beat until mixture is really stiff. Add more powdered sugar, and knead with your hands to create a nice, firm dough. Add some food coloring, and keep kneading to incorporate the color. Next, pour in about 15 drops of essential oil, or enough to get the flavor you want. Continue kneading to incorporate the flavor into the dough. Make dough balls with about one and a half teaspoons of the dough, and place onto a cookie sheet lined with parchment paper or waxed paper. Press balls flat with a fork, and let candies sit overnight to harden.

Chocolate Mint Bars   May 25

Materials

4-5 tbsp mashed dates
3 tbsp barley malt syrup
¾ C almond butter

3 tbsp cocoa
3-4 drops peppermint essential oil
1 C roasted almonds (optional)

Directions

Combine dates, barley malt, and peppermint essential oil. Add cashew butter and blend thoroughly. Add cocoa, and if nuts if you are using them. Shape mixture into bars, and refrigerate for a couple of hours before serving.

Springtime Chicken Bake   May 26

Materials

Small roasting chicken
3-4 tbsp extra virgin olive oil
2 drops rosemary essential oil
2 drops sage essential oil

2 drops lemon essential oil
1 small onion
Salt and pepper to taste

Directions

Cook the chicken with the onion, salt, and pepper. In a measuring cup, combine essential oils and olive oil. Brush oil mixture over chicken, and sprinkle some pepper on top. Return roaster to the oven and bake for an additional 15 minutes or so.

Hot Toddy for Adults   May 27

Materials

1 ounce whiskey
1 tbsp raw honey
1 bag lemon herbal tea

2-3 drops lemon essential oil
1 c boiling water

Directions

Combine water and herbal tea, and let steep for a couple of minutes. Remove the tea bag, and add the honey and lemon essential oil. Stir to mix, and drink to relieve a sore throat.

Dog Flea Shampoo   May 28

Materials

3 ounces liquid castile soap
1 ounce liquid aloe vera or aloe vera gel

10 drops sweet orange essential oil
10 drops cedarwood essential oil

Directions

Combine ingredients in a pump bottle. Shake to mix, and use regularly throughout flea and tick season.

Doggie Arthritis Treatment   May 29

Materials

2-3 tbsp vegetable oil or olive oil
3 drops rosemary essential oil

2 drops lavender essential oil
3 drops ginger essential oil

Directions

Combine essential oils and vegetable oils. To use, massage into dog's sore joints for pain relief. Take care to get right down to the skin beneath the fur.

Pregnancy Constipation Formula   May 30

Materials

1 tbsp rice bran oil

25-30 drops patchouli essential oil

Directions

Combine ingredients in a glass bowl. To use, rub on your belly in a clockwise motion to help combat constipation during pregnancy.

Hair Conditioning Treatment for Baldness   May 31

Materials

2 ml jojoba oil
2 drops palma rosa essential oil

2 drops geranium essential oil
6-8 drops evening primrose essential oil

Directions

Combine all ingredients in a glass bowl. To use, massage into scalp, and leave on for about a half an hour, and then rinse and shampoo as normal. Use weekly for the best results.

*U*SING AROMA THERAPY DIFFUSERS

Aroma therapy is a lot more than just filling your home with nice scents. You can use aroma therapy to improve your overall health, both physical and mental, and you don't need to do anything but inhale the scents. The easiest way to do this is to use an aroma therapy diffuser. When you combine various essential oils in the diffuser, the heat causes the vapors to rise and fill the room.

There are many different types of diffusers on the market, and there are even some essential oil blends that you can put right in your vaporizer. You can also make your own diffuser. Most diffusers work with tea light candles. All you need are candles, a flame-proof container to hold the candle, and a holder for the essential oils. If you use tea lights made with beeswax, you can enjoy up to eight hours of scents.

Essential Oil Blends

Throughout this book, you will find an assortment of essential oil blends to use in a diffuser. You can find hundreds more online, and there are several resources you can use that are loaded with information about aroma therapy essential oil blends. Once you get used to using essential oils and understand their various properties, you can start getting creative and come up with your own special blends, including holiday blends for parties.

The following are some of the most commonly-used essential oils for aroma therapy:

- Bergamot
- Cedarwood
- Chamomile
- Cinnamon
- Citronella
- Clove
- Coriander
- Eucalyptus
- Frankincense
- Geranium
- Grapefruit
- Jasmine
- Lavender
- Lemon
- Lime
- Mandarin
- Orange
- Peppermint
- Rose
- Sage
- Sandalwood
- Spearmint
- Tangerine
- Tea Tree
- Ylang-Ylang

June

The weather is getting warmer, and soon it will be time to hit the beach. Make sure that you are prepared, and have all of the skin care products you need to avoid damage from the harsh UV rays from the sun. This month, we have recipes for skin care, hair care, delicious treats, aromatherapy, and more. Always be sure to follow the exact recipes and not change the amount of essential oils, as some can cause reactions on those who have sensitive skin.

AROMATHERAPY BATH SALTS

Materials

1 C Epsom salts
2 C coarse sea salt
1 C baking soda
½ C citric acid

2 ½ tsp rice bran oil
30 drops lemon essential oil
30 drops orange essential oil

Directions

Mix dry ingredients in a glass bowl until there are no clumps. In a separate bowl, mix the essential oils. Add rice bran oil to the essential oils, and stir to blend. Add this mixture to the dry mixture, and blend well, using your hands. Store in a jar, tightly covered.

CHICKEN TAQUITOS

Materials

2 C shredded cooked chicken
½ C cream cheese
3 drops lime essential oil
¼ C salsa
1 tsp chili powder

1 tsp paprika
1 clove garlic, minced
1 onion, finely diced
1 C pepper jack cheese, grated
Flour tortillas

Directions

Preheat oven to 425 degrees. Combine softened cream cheese, salsa, chili powder, garlic, and lime essential oil in a glass boil. Stir to mix. Add chicken, onion, and cheese and mix well. Add about ¼ C of the mixture to the lower part of each tortilla, and roll up tortillas. Place tortillas seam side down on a greased baking sheet. Brush tops lightly with melted butter, or give them a shot of cooking spray. Bake for about 20 minutes, or until edges begin to turn golden brown. Serve with salsa and sour cream.

CREAM DEODORANT

Materials

¼ C baking soda
¼ C cornstarch

6 tbsp coconut oil
2-3 drops coconut essential oil for scent

Directions

Combine baking soda and cornstarch together in a glass boil. Add coconut oil, and stir with a fork until well blended. Add coconut essential oil. Store in a glass jar, cover, and label with the date.

*A*CNE CLAY MASK

June 4

Materials

2 ounces green clay
3 tsp corn flour
1 tsp water

1 drop chamomile essential oil
1 drop lavender essential oil
1 drop juniper essential oil

Directions

Follow the directions in the "Make Your Own Facial Clay Masks" section in this book.

*S*TICK DEODORANT

June 5

Materials

2 tbsp shea butter
3 tbsp coconut oil
2 tbsp corn starch

3 tbsp baking soda
3-4 drops lavender essential oil

Directions

In a double boiler over medium heat, combine shea butter and coconut oil until mixture just melts. Remove from heat, and add baking soda and corn starch. Mix well, and add the essential oils. Pour mixture into an old deodorant stick container and let harden over night.

*L*AVENDER SKIN TONIC

June 6

Materials

5 tbsp witch hazel
5 tbsp lemon juice, pulp removed

5 tbsp lavender water
3 drops lavender essential oil

Directions

Combine all of the ingredients into a dark colored glass bottle. Cover and shake. Remember to shake well every time you use it to ensure that the ingredients are thoroughly mixed.

*R*OSE BATH GEL

June 7

Materials

½ C water
¾ C grated castile soap
3 tbsp dried or fresh rose petals
3-4 drops rose essential oil

Directions

Crush the rose petals into a powder or paste (depending if you use dried or fresh flowers) with a mortar and pestle. Boil the water, and add the grated soap, stirring with a whisk until it is dissolved. Remove from heat, and add the rose essential oil and flower paste or powder. Pour into a glass bottle, cover, and label with the date.

Foamy Bath Oil   June 8

Materials

2 eggs
1 C extra virgin olive oil
1 C whole milk
2 tbsp raw honey
½ C corn oil

½ C almond oil
½ C vodka
1 tbsp unscented soap flakes
3 drops lavender essential oil

Directions

Combine eggs, oils, and honey in a glass bowl and beat well. Add milk, soap flakes, vodka, and essential oils, and continue beating until well blended. Store in covered bottles in the refrigerator. To use, add a tablespoon full under the tap runner when you are running a bath.

Sore Foot Soak   June 9

Materials

2 gallons warm water
3 drops peppermint essential oil

3 drops lavender essential oil
3 drops chamomile essential oil

Directions

Stir the essential oils into the warm water in a basin to use for soaking your feet. The peppermint essential oil will give your feet a tingle, and help to cool tired, hot, aching feet.

Athlete's Foot Soak   June 10

Materials

2 gallons warm water
4 drops tea tree oil

4 drops lavender essential oil
2 drops sandalwood essential oil

Directions

Add essential oils to the warm water in a basin for soaking feet. This mixture has anti-fungal properties with the tea tree oil and lavender essential oil, and the sandalwood will make your feet nice and soft.

Hand Soap

Materials

4 ounces liquid castile soap
20 drops lavender essential oil

10 drops rose essential oil
10 drops lemon essential oil

Directions

Combine castile soap and essential oils in a pump bottle. This is a great soap for softening your cuticles so you can easily push them back. It is also a disinfecting soap.

Brush-In Hair Scent

Materials

2 drops chamomile essential oil
2 drops lavender essential oil

2 drop sandalwood essential oil
½ ounce rice bran oil

Directions

Combine ingredients in a dark colored glass bottle. To use, apply a couple of drops to your brush or comb, and brush through your hair. Your hair will absorb the scent, and your scalp and hair will receive an extra conditioning treatment.

After-Sun Skin Re-Hydrator

Materials

1 tbsp jojoba oil
5 drops lavender essential oil

1 drop geranium essential oil
3 drops chamomile essential oil

Directions

Combine all of the ingredients into a glass bowl. To use, massage into your skin after it has been exposed to the harsh rays of the sun.

Focus Your Mind Room Spritz

Materials

3 ounces water
8-10 drops peppermint essential oil
6 drops rosemary essential oil

8 drops lime essential oil
2 drops lemon essential oil

Directions

Combine all of the ingredients into a spray bottle. To use, shake well, and spritz throughout any room in your house where you are going to be reading, studying, or doing anything else that involves concentration and focus.

FETA DIP

Materials

1 8 ounce package feta cheese
1 drop thyme essential oil
2 drops savory essential oil

1 drop lavender essential oil
2 cloves garlic

Directions

Combine all of the ingredients into a food processor, and blend until the mixture becomes a smooth paste. If it is too thick, add a bit of extra virgin olive oil to thin it out.

LAVENDER ROSE SOLID PERFUME

Materials

2 tsp grated beeswax
2 tsp rice bran oil

30 drops lavender essential oil
10 drops rose essential oil

Directions

In a double boiler over medium heat, melt the beeswax and rice bran oil together until they are blended. Remove from heat, and add essential oils. Quickly pour mixture into prepared containers, as it will harden fast. It will be ready to use in about 10 minutes or so.

WART TREATMENT

Materials

1 drop oregano essential oil
1 drop lemon essential oil

1 drop peppermint essential oil

Directions

Dilute the oregano essential oil in water, and apply one drop to the affected area. Next, apply the lemon essential oil, followed by the peppermint essential oil. Leave mixture on the wart, and put a band aid on top to keep it covered. Repeat twice daily until the wart is gone.

BRUISE TREATMENT

Materials

1 drop lavender essential oil

Directions

Apply lavender oil by a dropper right onto the bruise every 20 minutes until the pain starts to go away. This can also be used for cuts, insect bites, and mild burns.

Lavender Infused Lemonade

Materials

7-8 lemons
2-3 limes
1 gallon water

1 ½ C agave nectar
1 drop lavender essential oil

Directions

Squeeze the juice from the lemons and limes. Mix all of the ingredients into a glass pitcher, and refrigerate for a few hours. You can add more agave nectar if you want your lemonade to be sweeter. Serve over ice with a slice of lemon.

Carpet Freshener

Materials

30 drops cinnamon essential oil
30 drops eucalyptus essential oil
30 drops lemongrass essential oil

10 drops clove essential oil
½ C baking soda

Directions

Combine all of the ingredients in a shaker bottle, and set in a cool, dark place for 12-24 hours. To use, sprinkle over carpets, and let mixture sit for 15-20 minutes. Vacuum as normal.

Citrus Mint Room Spray

Materials

40 drops grapefruit essential oil
40 drops petit grain essential oil
40 drops peppermint essential oil

20 drops lime essential oil
10 drops lemon essential oil
½ C water

Directions

Combine all ingredients in a spray bottle. Shake well to mix, and shake well before each use.

Rheumatism Rub

Materials

1 ½ ounces rice bran oil
10 drops rosemary essential oil

7 drops lavender essential oil
8 drops juniper berry essential oil

Directions

Mix all of the ingredients together in a glass bottle and shake well before each use. To use, apply to the affected area and massage gently into the skin.

SORE MUSCLE MASSAGE OIL 1

Materials

1 ½ ounces rice bran oil
4 drops cinnamon essential oil

2 drops ginger essential oil
3 drops cajuput essential oil

Directions

Mix oils together and massage into your skin. This is a great oil to use on tired muscles after a workout.

SORE MUSCLE MASSAGE OIL 2

Materials

1 ½ ounces jojoba oil
4 drops cinnamon essential oil
3 drops chamomile essential oil

2 drops cajuput essential oil
6 drops allspice essential oil

Directions

Combine all of the ingredients and use like a regular massage oil. Like the previous recipe, this is another great oil to use after working out.

COLORED BATH SALTS

Materials

3 C Epsom salts
2 C baking soda
1 C coarse sea salt

Powdered food grade coloring
Essential oils (variety of your favorite scents)

Directions

Mix all of the ingredients together and store in glass jars. This makes a great gift, and you can layer colors and scents in the jars to make even prettier gifts, and tie a nice bow around the lid.

BODY DUSTING POWDER

Materials

¼ C corn starch
¾ C arrowroot powder

25 drops lavender essential oil

Directions

Combine all of the ingredients in a blender to mix thoroughly. Store in a covered container in a cool, dark place.

Softening Lip Balm

Materials

¼ C rice bran oil
¼ ounce shredded beeswax
1 tbsp liquid aloe vera

1 vitamin E capsule
10 drops lavender essential oil
5 drops sweet orange essential oil

Directions

In a double boiler over medium heat, combine beeswax and rice bran oil, and heat until they are melted together. Remove from heat, and add the essential oils, aloe vera, and liquid from the vitamin E capsule. Pour mixture into lip balm tubs. If you want to use tubes and have a more solid lip balm, simply add a bit more beeswax.

Almond/Oatmeal Facial Scrub

Materials

½ C raw almonds
½ C quick oats

10 drops lemongrass essential oil
15 drops lavender essential oil

Directions

Combine all of the dry ingredients in a blender and blend until they are well ground. Add the essential oils and mix. Use as you would a regular facial scrub.

Super-Insect Repellent

Materials

1 ounce pure distilled water
1 ounce liquid aloe vera
1 ounce witch hazel
5 drops tea tree oil
5 drops cinnamon leaf essential oil
6-8 drops lavender essential oil

8 drops frankincense essential oil
2 drops rosemary essential oil
2 drops rosewood essential oil
8 drops eucalyptus essential oil
7 drops clove bud essential oil
5 drops lemongrass essential oil

Directions

Combine all ingredients in a spray bottle. To use, shake well, and spray on clothing and exposed skin to keep the insects away. You can also spray this on outdoor furniture and other items that you want to keep the bugs off.

SUMMER PERFUME

Materials

2 drops rosemary essential oil
2 drops yarrow essential oil

2 drops lemongrass essential oil

Directions

Follow the directions in the "How to Make Your Own Perfumes Using Essential Oils" section of this book.

TIPS FOR COOKING WITH ESSENTIAL OILS

Many essential oils can take the place of the spices you use in many of your favorite recipes. While you should not use a large amount of essential oils, it is safe to consume them in small amounts. Here are some tips to help you create perfect meals, drinks, snacks, desserts, and more, using essential oils for flavoring.

Use Stronger Flavors – The best flavors to use are stronger ones, such as marjoram, nutmeg, oregano, thyme, basil, cinnamon, and peppermint. You only need about two drops to equal a two-ounce bottle of dried seasonings, so use the essential oils sparingly.

Don't Add Essential Oils while Cooking – The essential oils should be the last ingredients added, after the food has been cooked. This is because cooking will cause the oils to evaporate, and you will lose the flavors.

Dilute Essential Oils for Cooking – Because essential oils are so strong, it is a good idea to dilute them in olive oil, rice milk, almond milk, agave nectar, etc. before ingesting. For instance, if you are using one drop of oil, dilute it with one teaspoon of agave nectar, or two ounces of a drink. Do not give children under the age of two any foods that are made with essential oils.

Use Therapeutic-Grade Oils – When it comes to cooking with essential oils, be sure to only use oils that are therapeutic-grade. Read the label before using any essential oils to make sure that they are safe for cooking.

Do Not Use Your Microwave – Foods with essential oils should never be cooked in a microwave oven. All of the healthy enzymes in the essential oils will be completely destroyed after just a couple of seconds in the microwave, and harmful proteins could develop if you cook foods with essential oils in the microwave for 10 minutes or longer.

Do Not Use Sugar – Sugar can destroy the healthy enzymes in essential oils. If you need to use a sweetener, substitute sugar for agave nectar, fresh Stevia, or honey.

July

Now that summer is in full swing, you need to have protection from the hot sun. This month, we will have some sun lotion recipes, along with recipes for after-sun skin care. Of course, there will be plenty of other great recipes for you to try as well, including refreshing drinks, more skin care, pet care, perfumes, and aroma therapy.

After-Sun Aloe Vera Gel July 1

Materials

8 tbsp aloe vera gel
6 drops chamomile essential oil

8 drops lavender essential oil

Directions

Pour the aloe vera gel into a pump bottle, and add the essential oils. Shake well to mix. Label with the date, and store in the fridge for a cooling sunburn relief.

Soothing Sunburn Lotion July 2

Materials

8 tbsp plain yogurt
1 small cucumber

8 drops lavender essential oil

Directions

Put the cucumber in a juicer and extract enough juice for 4 tablespoons. Mix this juice with the yogurt, and then add the essential oils. Smooth over all of the affected areas of your skin, and let the mixture sit on the skin for around 15 minutes. Rinse with lukewarm water and pat dry.

Sunscreen Lotion Bars July 3

Materials

5 tbsp shredded beeswax or pellets
½ C shea butter
½ C coconut oil
2 vitamin E capsules

2 tbsp zinc oxide
5-6 drops lemon essential oil (for scent, and as an insect repellant)

Directions

In a double boiler over medium heat, combine shea butter, coconut oil, and beeswax. When ingredients are melted and mixed together, remove from heat. Stir in zinc oxide, and then add the essential oils and the liquid from the vitamin E capsule. Pour into soap mold and let set. Store in an airtight container. These bars will melt in the sun, so apply to skin before going outside, or just take a small piece with you in an airtight container.

Cherry Lemonade

Materials

1 C agave nectar
2 drops lemon essential oil
4-5 lemons

2 C sour cherry juice
1 quart soda water or sparkling mineral water

Directions

Combine agave nectar, juice from lemons, sour cherry juice, and lemon essential oil and stir. Add sparkling water. Chill before serving and serve with ice and lemon wedges.

Peppermint Iced Tea

July 5

Materials

4 green tea bags
¼ C agave nectar
3-4 drops peppermint essential oil

3 limes
4 C boiling water
Mint sprigs

Directions

Pour agave nectar and peppermint essential oil into a glass juice pitcher. Cover with boiling water and stir. Add tea bags, and allow mixture to steep until it is a nice, dark color. Serve with ice, lime wedges, and a sprig of mint.

Happiness Perfume

July 6

Materials

1 drop jasmine essential oil
1 drop rose essential oil

2 drops sandalwood essential oil
2 drops sweet orange essential oil

Directions

Follow the directions in the "How to Make Your Own Perfumes Using Essential Oils" section in this book.

Coconut Body Scrub

July 7

Materials

5 tbsp Epsom salts
1 tbsp coconut oil
8 drops lime essential oil
6 drops ylang ylang essential oil

Directions

Combine Epsom salts and coconut oil and mix well. Add the essential oils and mix well. Store in a glass jar, cover, and label with the date. Use on your entire body, particularly on any rough patches. Do not use this mixture on your face or other sensitive parts of the body.

Mature Skin Clay Mask   July 8

Materials

1 ounce red clay
3 tbsp rosewater
2 tsp oatmeal, finely ground
1 tsp rice bran oil

2 drops rose essential oil
1 drop neroli essential oil
1 drop frankincense essential oil

Directions

Follow the directions in the "How to Make Clay Facial Masks with Essential Oils" section in this book.

Relaxation Diffuser Blend   July 9

Materials

2 drops chamomile essential oil
2 drops lavender essential oil

2 drops marjoram essential oil

Directions

Follow the instructions in the "Using Aroma Therapy Diffusers" section of this book.

Brain Power Diffuser Blend   July 10

Materials

2 drops rosemary essential oil
4 drops coriander essential oil

2 drops black pepper essential oil

Directions

Follow the instructions in the "Using Aroma Therapy Diffusers" section of this book.

Bath Fizz   July 11

Materials

1 C bicarbonate of soda
½ C citric acid
½ tsp red clay

20 drops orange essential oil

Directions

Mix all of the ingredients and press into molds or muffin tins. Allow to sit overnight, remove from tins, and store in airtight containers until you are ready to use them. Depending on the size, put one or two into your bath water.

Conditioning Hair Oil July 12

Materials

½ ounce jojoba oil
2 drops chamomile essential oil
2 drops sandalwood essential oil

2 drops lavender essential oil
2 drops jasmine essential oil

Directions

Combine all ingredients and massage into hair and scalp. Let sit for 30-60 minutes, rinse, and shampoo as normal.

Scented Foot Powder July 13

Materials

¼ C baking soda
1/8 C corn starch
1/8 C clay

4 drops grapefruit essential oil
4 drops pine essential oil

Directions

Combine baking soda, corn starch, clay, and essential oil, making sure that there are no lumps. Store in an airtight container, cover, and label with the date.

Foot Bath July 14

Materials

2 gallons warm water
5 drops lemon essential oil

4 drops lavender essential oil
2 drops rosemary essential oil

Directions

Add essential oils to warm water in a foot basin, and stir to mix. Soak for a half an hour, or until the water begins to cool down.

Clay Mask for Normal Skin

Materials

3 tsp corn flour
2 ounces green clay
1 egg yolk

1 tsp pure distilled water
1 drop of a mix of 2 drops geranium
essential oil and 1 drop rose essential oil

Directions

Follow the instructions in the "How to Make Clay Facial Masks with Essential Oils" section in this book.

Dry Skin Clay Facial Mask

Materials

3 tsp corn flour
2 ounces green clay
1 egg yolk
1 tsp evening primrose oil

1 drop carrot essential oil
1 drop of a mixture of 1 drop chamomile
essential oil and 1 drop rose essential oil
2 tsp pure distilled water

Directions

Follow the instructions in the "How to Make Clay Facial Masks with Essential Oils" section in this book.

Oily Skin Clay Facial Mask

Materials

3 tsp corn flour
2 ounces green clay
1 tbsp Brewer's yeast

1 tbsp pure distilled water
1 drop lavender essential oil
1 drop rosemary essential oil

Directions

Follow the instructions in the "How to Make Clay Facial Masks with Essential Oils" section in this book.

Sunscreen Bar

Materials

1 C coconut oil
1 C cocoa butter
1 ¼ C shredded beeswax

2 tbsp zinc oxide powder
2 vitamin E capsules
2 drops lavender essential oil

Directions

In a double boiler over medium heat, combine coconut oil, cocoa butter, beeswax, and the liquid from the vitamin E capsules. Stir constantly until the ingredients are melted and blended together. Remove from heat, and add essential oils and zinc oxide powder. Stir to mix. Pour into molds and allow to cool. Remove from molds, and store in airtight containers.

*I*NSECT REPELLENT BAR **July 19**

Materials

1 C coconut oil
¼ C shea butter
¼ C cocoa butter
½ C plus 2 tbsp shredded beeswax
¼ C rosemary leaves (fresh or dried)
1 tsp whole cloves
2 tsp thyme (fresh or dried)

1 tsp ground cinnamon
¼ C dried catnip leaf
1 tbsp mint leaf
2 vitamin E capsules
10 drops lemon essential oil
10 drops lavender essential oil
10 drops eucalyptus essential oil

Directions

In a double boiler over medium heat, combine rosemary, cloves, thyme, cinnamon, catnip, mint, and coconut oil. Cover, and heat for 30 minutes, or until the oil is darker in color and you can really smell the rosemary. Strain the dried herbs from the oil, and put the oil back into the double boiler. This mixture is going to reduce, and you will end up with about ½ C of the oil when you are finished. Add butters and beeswax. When the mixture has melted, remove from heat and add the liquid from the vitamin E capsule and essential oils. Pour mixture into molds and let sit overnight to harden.

*U*PLIFTING PERFUME **July 20**

Materials

3 drops lavender essential oil
5 drops tangerine essential oil
2 drops orange essential oil

1 drop ylang ylang essential oil
2 drops clary sage essential oil
1 tsp fragrance oil

Directions

Follow the instructions in the "How to Make Your Own Perfumes Using Essential Oils" section in this book.

*I*NTESTINAL AILMENT BLEND **July 21**

Materials

1 drop chamomile essential oil
1 drop peppermint essential oil
2 drops rosemary essential oil

1 drop clove essential oil
1 tsp rice bran oil

Directions

Combine all of the ingredients, and rub onto your belly where you are feeling pain or discomfort.

Multi-Purpose Cleaner July 22

Materials

2 C vinegar
2 C water

5 drops lemon essential oil
10 drops pine essential oil

Directions

Combine ingredients in a spray bottle and shake well. To use, shake before using, and spray onto hard surfaces that need cleaning. This can also be used as a floor cleaner, but it may be damaging to some wood floors, so test s small section first.

Flea and Tick Repellent July 23

Materials

½ tsp alcohol
1 drop cedarwood essential oil
3 drops purification essential oil
3 drops lavender essential oil

3 drops citronella essential oil
1 drop thyme essential oil
2 drops orange essential oil

Directions

Combine all ingredients, and massage into dog's fur.

Wrinkle Cream July 24

Materials

2 ounces jojoba oil
5 drops lavender essential oil
5 drops rose essential oil

5 drops geranium essential oil
5 drops rosemary essential oil

Directions

Combine all of the ingredients, and pour into a glass jar. Cover, and label with the date. For best results, use twice daily, in the morning and in the evening.

Glowing Skin Exfoliate July 25

Materials

¼ C Kosher salt
¼ C coarse sea salt
¼ C Epsom salts
2 ounces jojoba oil

10 drops lemon essential oil
5 drops rosemary essential oil
5 drops mint essential oil

Directions

Mix all of the ingredients together in a glass bowl. Store in glass jars. To use, apply to skin and massage in to exfoliate. Rinse with clear, warm water.

ROMANTIC MASSAGE OIL   July 26

Materials

1 ounce extra virgin olive oil   10 drops lavender essential oil
20 drops rose essential oil

Directions

Mix ingredients in a glass bowl. If not using right away, store in a dark glass bottle in a cool, dark place.

SORE JOINT OIL   July 27

Materials

1 C extra virgin olive oil   4 drops cajuput essential oil
8 drops eucalyptus essential oil   1 drop black pepper essential oil
8 drops marjoram essential oil

Directions

Mix all of the ingredients in a glass jar and shake well to mix. Warm mixture in your hands before massaging onto affected areas.

AIR FRESHENING SPRAY   July 28

Materials

25 drops spearmint essential oil   20 drops clove bud essential oil
25 drops sage essential oil   4 ounces pure distilled water
20 drops marjoram essential oil

Directions

Mix all of the ingredients in a spray bottle. Shake well before each use.

CARPET FRESHENER   July 29

Materials

½ C baking soda   25 drops eucalyptus essential oil
25 drops lemongrass essential oil   35 drops cinnamon leaf essential oil
15 drops clove bud essential oil

Directions

Blend all of the ingredients in a jar. Cover, and let sit for 24-48 hours. To use, sprinkle on carpets, allow to sit for about 15 minutes, and then vacuum as normal.

Pet Odor Diffuser Blend   July 30

Materials

8 drops lavender essential oil
15 drops orange essential oil
6 drops lemon essential oil

5 drops tea tree oil
5 drops geranium essential oil
2 drops neroli essential oil

Directions

Follow the instructions in the "Using Aroma Therapy Diffusers" section of this book.

Citrus Popsicles   July 31

Materials

2 quarts of water
2 drops grapefruit essential oil
2 drops lime essential oil

2 drops lemon essential oil
2 drops orange essential oil
2 drops tangerine essential oil

Directions

Combine all ingredients in a glass bowl or pitcher. Pour into popsicle molds, and freeze overnight. This can also be used as a delicious and refreshing drink.

MAKE SOLID PERFUME WITH ESSENTIAL OILS

Solid perfumes are nice, because you can apply them in more specific areas of your body than you can with a spray. This type of perfume is easy to make, and you don't need to go out and buy any special tools. All you need are the ingredients for your specific recipe, which will include beeswax, carrier oil, and up to 50 drops of essential oils, and of course, some pretty tins to store your perfume in.

How to Do It

The first step is to blend the essential oils. You may want to play around with different blends to find something that suits you perfectly. Once you have done this, it is time to start making the solid perfume. Measure the carrier oil as per the recipe you are using. In a double boiler over medium heat, melt the beeswax with the carrier oil. When they are combined, remove from heat and add the essential oils. You have to work fast, because the beeswax will harden quickly. As soon as everything is blended, pour or spoon mixture into prepared tins.

Presentation Ideas

Solid perfumes are a great gift idea, and there are so many ways that you can present them as gifts. Of course, the most important part of the presentation is the tin, and there are several options. You can search through antique stores and flea markets to find old tins that have lots of character. You can also use old candy tins, or buy tins at your local dollar store or craft store. If you are using old or undecorated tins, you may want to paint designs on them, add rhinestones and bows, and tie with a ribbon.

August

There is still lots of time left for barbecues and outdoor summer parties, and this month, we have some fun recipes for your parties, including slow cooker recipes that involve almost no work at all. You will also find skin and hair care recipes, as well as acne formulas for teens to help them get ready to go back to school next month. Look for more household products that will leave your home smelling fresh and clean, and of course, perfumes and aroma therapy recipes.

Slow Cooker Meatballs

Materials

2 lbs ground beef
2 large eggs
1 lb ground pork
3 tbsp coconut flour
1/3 C grated parmesan cheese

3 cloves garlic, minced
2 drops fennel essential oil
1 tsp sea salt
3 C home-made pasta sauce

Directions

Combine all of the ingredients except for the pasta sauce in a large bowl. Blend well with your hands to make sure that the ingredients are well blended. Form into meatballs (about 1 ½ inches across). Add sauce to the slow cooker, and then add the meatballs. Cook on high for 3-4 hours.

Home-Made Pasta Sauce

Materials

5-6 plum tomatoes, seeds removed
2 cans tomato paste
2 cloves garlic, minced
2 tbsp white sugar
1 tsp ground black pepper

1 drop clove essential oil
1 tsp paprika
1 tsp chili powder
1 tsp cayenne pepper

Directions

Put tomatoes in a food processor, and mix until they are liquefied. The skins will shred, and then liquefy during the cooking process. Add the tomato paste, sugar, garlic, spices, and clove essential oil. Cook in the slow cooker on low for 6-8 hours.

Shower Gel

Materials

2/3 C liquid castile soap
2 tbsp raw honey
2 vitamin E capsules
1 tsp jojoba oil

2 tsp vegetable glycerin
10 drops lemon essential oil
5 drops grapefruit essential oil

Directions

Combine all of the ingredients in a glass bowl, and whisk to blend. Pour into a pump bottle, and use whenever you want a fresh scent in the shower.

MOOD ENHANCING PERFUME

August 4

Materials

1 drop ylang ylang essential oil
1 drop bergamot essential oil
3 drops clary sage essential oil

4 drops lavender essential oil
3 drops tangerine essential oil

Directions

Follow the instructions in the "How to Make Your Own Perfumes Using Essential Oils" section of this book.

ATHLETE'S FOOT/RINGWORM TREATMENT

August 5

Materials

2 drops tea tree essential oil
1 drop lavender essential oil

1 tsp grape seed oil

Directions

Combine ingredients in a small glass bowl, stirring to mix. To use, apply to affected area with a cotton swab.

BURN TREATMENT

August 6

Materials

2 drops lavender essential oil

Directions

When you have a minor burn, apply the lavender essential oil to the affected area for relief.

BED-TIME AROMA THERAPY

August 7

Materials

3 drops ho wood essential oil
3 drops ylang ylang essential oil

3 drops bergamot essential oil

Directions

Follow the instructions in the "Using Aroma Therapy Diffusers" section in this book.

Facial Cleanser

Materials

2 ounces pure distilled water
1 drop marshmallow essential oil
1 drop chamomile essential oil

1 drop olive leaf essential oil
1 drop rose hip essential oil

Directions

Combine all of the ingredients in a small glass bowl, and stir to mix. To use, dip a sponge into the mixture, and rub on your face for exfoliation, followed by pouring the rest of the mixture onto a washcloth and washing your whole face and neck area.

Foaming Facial Cleanser

Materials

4 tbsp liquid castile soap
3 tsp avocado oil
4 drops lemon essential oil

4 drops orange essential oil
4 drops grapefruit essential oil

Directions

Combine all of the ingredients together in a glass bottle. Cover and store in a cool, dark place. Shake well before each use.

Shaving Cream

Materials

1 small cucumber
1 C cocoa butter
4 tbsp almond oil
2 tbsp avocado oil

3 tbsp witch hazel
5 drops lavender essential oil
2 drops carrot essential oil

Directions

Place the cucumber in a juicer so you get 1 tbsp of juice. In a double boiler over medium heat, melt the cocoa butter. Remove from heat, and add the almond oil, avocado oil, and witch hazel. Stir to mix, and add the cucumber juice and essential oils. Pour into a glass jar, cover, and label with the date. Store for up to two weeks in the refrigerator.

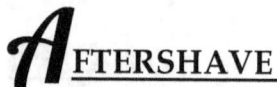FTERSHAVE

Materials

2 tbsp pure distilled water
2 tbsp witch hazel
3 tbsp alcohol
1 tbsp vegetable glycerin

10 drops bay essential oil
10 drops cinnamon essential oil
12 drops coriander essential oil
15 drops orange essential oil

Directions

Mix 1 tbsp of alcohol and essential oils in a glass jar. In a second jar, add the rest of the alcohol, distilled water, witch hazel, and glycerin, and mix well. Slowly add the essential oil mixture to the water mixture. Pour into a dark colored glass bottle. Cover, label with the date, and store in a cool, dark place for up to two weeks.

Elbow Cream

Materials

1 tbsp grated beeswax
¼ C avocado oil
¼ C cocoa butter
1 vitamin E capsule

1 tbsp rosewater
3 drops lavender essential oil
4 drops orange essential oil
1 drop carrot essential oil

Directions

In a double boiler over medium heat, combine the beeswax, avocado oil, and cocoa butter. Heat until the ingredients are melted and blended together, and add the liquid from the vitamin E capsule. Heat the rosewater in another double boiler, and slowly add half of it to the oil mixture. Remove from heat, and continue to add the rosewater. As the mixture thickens, add the essential oils and stir with a whisk. Pour into glass jars, cover, and label with the date.

Eye Tonic

Materials

1 C rosewater
1 tsp castor oil

2 tbsp cornflower petals
1 drop rose essential oil

Directions

Chop up the cornflower petals, and put them in a saucepan with the rosewater. Simmer for 15-20 minutes. Add castor oil and rose essential oil. Pour into a glass jar, cover, and shake to mix the ingredients. Label with the date. To use, soak cotton balls or pads in the tonic, place over your eyes, and sit quietly for 10-15 minutes. Store in the refrigerator to make the mixture more revitalizing.

Aloe Vera Face Gel for Dry Skin

Materials

8 tbsp aloe vera gel
4 drops carrot essential oil

3 drops chamomile essential oil
3 drops sandalwood essential oil

Directions

Combine ingredients into a clean jar. Cover, shake well to mix, and label with the date. To use, apply a small amount of the gel to your face and neck, and massage into the skin. Rinse with warm water and pat dry.

Aloe Vera Face Gel for Problem Skin

Materials

4 tbsp aloe vera gel
3 drops geranium essential oil

2 drops parsley essential oil
3 drops carrot essential oil

Directions

Combine ingredients into a clean jar. Cover, shake well to mix, and label with the date. To use, apply a small amount of the gel to your face and neck, and massage into the skin. Rinse with warm water and pat dry.

Aloe Vera Face Gel for Acne

Materials

4 tbsp aloe vera gel
4 drops lavender essential oil

2 drops tea tree oil
2 drops juniper essential oil

Directions

Combine ingredients into a clean jar. Cover, shake well to mix, and label with the date. To use, apply a small amount of the gel to your face and neck, and massage into the skin. Rinse with warm water and pat dry.

Acne Treatment

Materials

3 tbsp jojoba oil
6 drops lavender essential oil
3 drops tea tree oil
2 drops geranium essential oil

Directions

Combine all of the ingredients in a dark colored glass bottle. Shake well. To use, shake to mix ingredients, and apply to affected areas on clean skin twice each day.

MORNING SHOWER GEL   August 18

Materials

1 C shower gel base
10 drops geranium essential oil
10 drops bergamot essential oil
6 drops rosemary essential oil

5 drops juniper essential oil
5 drops petit grain essential oil
2 drops basil essential oil

Directions

Combine ingredients in a glass bowl, stirring gently to mix without creating any bubbles. Add some food grade colorant if you want. Pour mixture into a pump bottle, and use in your morning showers.

SOFT LIPS BALM   August 19

Materials

2 tbsp grated beeswax
1 tbsp cocoa butter
4 tbsp rice bran oil

1 tsp carrot-infused oil
5 drops spearmint essential oil

Directions

In a double boiler over medium heat, combine beeswax, cocoa butter, and rice bran oil. Heat until ingredients are melted and blended together, and add the carrot-infused oil. Mix well. When mixture begins to cool, add the spearmint essential oil. Pour mixture into prepared lip balm tubs or tubes.

HAND OIL   August 20

Materials

1 tsp raw honey
2 tbsp jojoba oil
2 tsp rice bran oil

1 tbsp rosewater
8 drops lemon essential oil

Directions

In a double boiler over medium heat, combine honey, rice bran oil, and jojoba oil. Heat until ingredients are melted and blended together. Heat the rosewater in another double boiler. Slowly add half of the heated rosewater to the oil mixture, and remove from heat. Continue adding the rosewater, and stir with a whisk. Add the lemon essential oil, stir, and pour into a glass jar. Cover and label with the date.

Neck Cream

Materials

1 tbsp grated beeswax
¼ C rice bran oil
¼ C wheat germ oil
1 vitamin E capsule

1 tbsp chamomile water
2 drops geranium essential oil
5 drops chamomile essential oil
2 drops lemon essential oil

Directions

In a double boiler over medium heat, combine beeswax, rice bran oil, and wheat germ oil. Heat until ingredients are melted and blended together, and add the liquid from the vitamin E capsule. Heat the chamomile water in another double boiler. Slowly add half of the heated chamomile water to the oil mixture. Remove from heat, and add the rest of the chamomile water. Stir with a whisk. As the mixture begins to thicken, add the essential oils and stir to mix. Pour into a glass jar, cover, and label with the date.

Acne Face Mask

Materials

1 ounce green clay
3 tbsp aloe vera gel
1 tsp orange flower water

1 drop orange essential oil
1 drop lavender essential oil
1 drop tea tree oil

Directions

Follow the instructions in the "How to Make Clay Masks with Essential Oils" section of this book.

Peaceful Perfume

Materials

2 drops clary sage essential oil
2 drops cypress essential oil

4 drops bergamot essential oil

Directions

Follow the instructions in the "How to Make Your Own Perfumes Using Essential Oils" section of this book.

Family Room Diffuser Blend

Materials

1 drop sandalwood essential oil

3 drops lavender essential oil

Directions

Follow the instructions in the "Using Aroma Therapy Diffusers" section of this book.

LAVENDER BATH FIZZ

Materials

1 C baking soda
½ C citric acid

1 tbsp cocoa butter
15-20 drops lavender essential oil

Directions

Combine all of the ingredients together, and pack into molds. Let sit overnight to harden, and then use 1-2 pieces in your bathwater.

DANDRUFF HAIR OIL

Materials

½ ounce sweet almond oil
2 drops cedarwood essential oil
2 drops lavender essential oil

2 drops rosemary essential oil
2 drops tea tree oil

Directions

Mix all of the ingredients, and massage into your scalp. Rinse with warm water, and shampoo as normal.

REVITALIZING FACIAL MASK

Materials

2 ounces green clay
3 tsp corn flour
1 egg yolk
1 tsp Brewer's yeast
1 tsp jojoba oil

1 tbsp pure distilled water
2 drops carrot essential oil
1 drop chamomile essential oil
1 drop lavender essential oil

Directions

Follow the instructions in the "How to Make Clay Facial Masks with Essential Oils" section of this book.

CITRUS ROOM SPRITZ

Materials

3 ounces pure distilled water

15 drops lemon essential oil

Directions

Combine ingredients into a spray bottle. Shake before using.

CITRUS BODY SPRAY

Materials

4 ounces witch hazel
5 drops sweet orange essential oil

3 drops grapefruit essential oil
5 drops lemon essential oil

Directions

Combine all of the ingredients into a pump spray bottle, and shake well to mix. Store in the refrigerator for up to two weeks, shaking well before each use.

SEA SALT FACIAL SCRUB

Materials

1 C coarse sea salt
1 tbsp liquid aloe vera

1 vitamin E capsule
2 drops chamomile essential oil

Directions

Combine sea salt, liquid aloe vera, the liquid from the vitamin E capsule, and chamomile essential oil together in a glass bowl. Store in a covered glass jar. To use, apply 2 tbsp of the mixture to your face, and massage into skin. Rinse with clear, warm water.

TEMPLE MASSAGE OIL

Materials

1 tbsp rice bran oil
3 drops clary sage essential oil

3 drops bergamot essential oil

Directions

Combine all of the ingredients together in a small glass bottle. Use 1-2 drops to massage into your temples, and sit back and relax for 15-20 minutes.

ESSENTIAL OILS AND PREGNANCY

There are many unwanted symptoms that go along with pregnancy, and unfortunately, it is not always safe to take medications for those symptoms. Luckily, there are many essential oils that are perfectly safe for pregnant women to use, and that will help ease a lot of those nasty symptoms. Using a diffuser is a great way for pregnant women to get the benefits of essential oils, and this is perfectly safe at any stage of your pregnancy. To be on the safe side, just like you would with any medication, be sure to discuss using essential oils with your doctor before you begin.

Essential Oils can be Beneficial to Pregnant Women

Once your doctor gives you the okay to use certain essential oils, you will find that there are many benefits to using them. They can help to treat a number of pregnancy symptoms, including swollen ankles, nausea, and general aches and pains. They can also help you to relax and feel calmer, or give you energy when you need it and even increase your power of concentration.

Which Essential Oils Can You Use during Pregnancy?

While not all essential oils are safe to use during pregnancy, there are several that you can use daily, or even several times a day. For instance, orange is a great oil to use any time, and it will help you to feel relaxed and happy. Ylang ylang is another good one to have on hand when you are pregnant, because it can help to keep your blood pressure regulated, and it is good for tension. Another essential oil that can help with tension and nerves is neroli. Here are some more essential oils that are beneficial during pregnancy.

Eucalyptus – Rather than take an over-the-counter medication for congestion, this essential oil will work just as well, and is safer during pregnancy.

Tea Tree Oil – If you experience thrush during pregnancy, tea tree oil can help.

Cypress – After you are five months along, you can use this essential oil to help relieve swollen ankles.

Sandalwood – Use this essential oil to help you relax or sleep. It is also good for treating cycstitis.

Geranium – This is an essential oil that is going to help you to have more energy, as well as better circulation.

During pregnancy, avoid using the following essential oils: almond; basil; black pepper; cedarwood; chamomile; cinnamon; clove; fennel; myrhh; lemongrass; lemon; horseradish; jasmine; rosemary; oregano; stinging nettle; sage; pine; nutmeg; peppermint; rose; and thyme.

September

The kids are back to school, and fall will soon be here. The weather will start to get cooler, and that is going to affect your skin. This month, we have all kinds of great skin care recipes using essential oils that will keep your skin from becoming dried out in the cool fall air. Of course, there are also loads of other recipes, including delicious foods, aroma therapy, perfumes, and more.

Disinfecting Bathroom Diffuser Blend

Materials

4 drops pine essential oil
2 drops thyme essential oil

3 drops eucalyptus essential oil

Directions

Follow the instructions in the "Using Aroma Therapy Diffusers" section of this book.

Rose Bath Fizz

Materials

1 C baking soda
½ C citric acid
3 tbsp rose petals

5 drops rose essential oil
10 drops rose geranium essential oil
3 drops rosewood essential oil

Directions

Combine all of the ingredients. Mix well, and press into molds and let sit overnight to harden. To use, place one or two pieces in your bath water.

Scalp Massage Oil

Materials

½ ounce sweet almond oil
2 drops rosemary essential oil
2 drops lavender essential oil

1 drop clary sage essential oil
1 drop jasmine essential oil

Directions

Combine all of the ingredients together and pour into a dark glass bottle (amber is preferable as it doesn't allow light to get in). To use, put 4-5 drops of the oil mixture onto your fingertips, and massage into your scalp. Allow to sit for 5-10 minutes, then rinse and shampoo as normal.

Essential Oil Shampoo

Materials

1 tbsp sweet almond oil
3 drops lavender essential oil
2 drops rose essential oil

1 drop lemon essential oil
Shampoo of choice

Directions

Combine the first four ingredients, and pour into a dark glass bottle (amber to keep the light out). Add 7-8 drops of this mixture to your favorite shampoo.

Anti-Fungal Foot Soak

September 5

Materials

5 drops tea tree oil
3 drops peppermint essential oil

Basin filled with hot water

Directions

Fill basin with water as hot as you can stand soaking in. Add the essential oils, and stir to mix. Soak feet until water starts to get cool.

Purifying Facial Mask

September 6

Materials

2 ounces green clay
3 tsp cornflour
1 egg yolk

1 drop carrot essential oil
1 drop rose essential oil

Directions

Mix all of the ingredients together to form a paste. To use, apply to skin on face and neck, and let sit for 15-20 minutes. Rinse with clear, warm water, and pat skin dry.

Citrus Bathroom Spray

September 7

Materials

4 drops lemon essential oil
4 drops lime essential oil

3 drops orange essential oil
2 ounces witch hazel extract

Directions

Combine all of the ingredients in a small spray bottle. To use, shake well, and spray when you need a fresh, citrus scent in the bathroom. This can also be used as a dusting spray, and will leave a fresh scent throughout your home.

Sore Muscle Rub

September 8

Materials

15 drops marjoram essential oil
20 drops lemongrass essential oil
8 drops sandalwood essential oil
10 drops lavender essential oil

10 drops cypress essential oil
10 drops deep blue essential oil
rice bran oil

Directions

Combine all essential oils together and pour into a roller bottle, and top up with rice bran oil. To use, apply to affected area when you have ligament, muscle, and joint pain.

$\mathcal{H}$EADACHE RUB   September 9

Materials

30 drops peppermint essential oil
15 drops wintergreen essential oil
20 drops lavender essential oil

10 drops birch essential oil
5 drops frankincense essential oil
Rice bran oil

Directions

Combine all of the essential oils in a roller bottle, and top up with rice bran oil. To use, apply to your temples, forehead, and back of the neck.

$\mathcal{K}$IDS' AROMA THERAPY FOR COLDS   September 10

Materials

8 drops eucalyptus essential oil
10 drops ravensara essential oil
5 drops tea tree oil

3 drops lavender essential oils
1 drop thyme essential oil
2 drops peppermint essential oil

Directions

Mix all of the essential oils in a dark glass bottle (amber is preferable to keep the light out). To use, for babies 2-18 months, mix 1 drop of oil mixture with 1 tsp vegetable oil, and add to bath water. For babies 18 months-3 years, add 2 drops of oil mixture. For children ages 3-6 years, add 3 drops of oil mixture. For children 7-11 years, add 4 drops of oil mixture. For children 12 and older, add 5 drops of oil mixture.

$\mathcal{E}$XFOLIATING FOOT SCRUB   September 11

Materials

¼ C coarse sea salt
¼ C sweet almond oil

15 drops peppermint essential oil

Directions

Combine all of the ingredients, and store in a covered glass jar. To use, place a small amount of the mixture onto the palm of your hand, and rub all over moistened skin. Rinse in the shower, being careful because the oils can be slippery.

$\mathcal{R}$ELAXING MASSAGE OIL   September 12

Materials

1 ounce pure vegetable oil
5 drops Roman chamomile essential oil

5 drops jasmine essential oil
5 drops lavender essential oil

Directions

Combine all of the ingredients in a dark glass bottle (amber is best because it doesn't allow light to get in). Cover, and label with the date. To use, apply a couple of drops to the skin and massage gently.

Woodsy Air Freshener   September 13

Materials

4 ounces pure distilled water
70 drops pine essential oil

30 drops cedarwood essential oil
20 drops juniper berry essential oil

Directions

Combine all of the ingredients in a spray bottle. To use, shake well, and mist into the air.

Air Purifying Aroma Therapy   September 14

Materials

20 drops clove essential oil
25 drops lemon essential oil
15 drops cinnamon bark essential oil

5 drops eucalyptus essential oil
5 drops rosemary essential oil

Directions

Combine all of the ingredients into a dark colored glass bottle (amber is best as it doesn't allow light to get in and ruin the effects of the essential oils). To use, follow the instructions in the "Using Aroma Therapy Diffusers" section of this book.

Chicken Noodle Soup   September 15

Materials

1 tbsp coconut oil
1 drop thyme essential oil
1 drop sage essential oil
2 cloves garlic, minced
1 medium onion, chopped

2 celery stalks, chopped
6-8 C chicken broth
1-2 C egg noodles
2 C diced cooked chicken
Salt and pepper to taste

Directions

In a large saucepan, combine coconut oil, celery, onion, and chicken. Cook over medium-low heat for 3 minutes, and then add garlic. Cook for another 2-3 minutes. Add broth, salt, and pepper, and turn heat up to medium. Bring to a boil, and add egg noodles. Cook for 10 minutes or so until noodles are tender, add thyme essential oil, remove from heat, and serve.

Cinnamon Milk

Materials

¾ C raw almonds
3 C soft dates, pitted
4 C water

1 drop cinnamon essential oil
3 drops orange essential oil

Directions

Soak almonds and dates in a couple of cups of water for 12 hours. Add remaining water and mix until smooth. Add essential oils. Strain mixture through a sieve to get rid of any lumps of dates or almonds, and then chill in the refrigerator.

Fruit Dip

Materials

1 bag mini marshmallows
1 8-ounce package softened cream cheese

2 drops sweet orange essential oil

Directions

Combine all of the ingredients in a glass bowl, and serve with slices of fruit, grapes, melon balls, etc.

Citrus Floor Cleaner

Materials

10 drops sweet orange essential oil
5 drops lemon essential oil

1 gallon hot water

Directions

Combine essential oils in a bucket of hot water. Clean floors as normal. Rinse with clear water to get rid of any oily residue.

Kitchen Pest Control

Materials

Peppermint, eucalyptus, or citronella essential oil, or a combination of these oils

Directions

Apply 15-20 drops or oil in areas around your home that are damp or moist, including plumbing fixtures, basements, and the garage.

Dog Earwax Treatment

Materials

1 tsp witch hazel

3 drops lavender essential oil

Directions

Combine ingredients and store in a dark colored glass bottle (amber is best in order to keep light out). To use, apply 4 drops of the mixture into your dog's ear canal, or soak a cotton ball with the mixture and massage the ear. Repeat daily.

Kitty Flea Collar

Materials

½ tsp rubbing alcohol
1 drop cedarwood essential oil
1 drop lavender essential oil

1 drop citronella essential oil
4 garlic capsules

Directions

Combine alcohol, essential oils, and the powder from the garlic capsules in a glass bowl. Apply mixture to your cat's collar, and allow it to dry before putting in the cat. Add a new mixture to the collar every month or so.

Hair Loss Oil Treatment

Materials

4 drops rosemary essential oil
4 drops geranium essential oil
3 drops lavender essential oil
3 drops cypress essential oil

1 drop frankincense essential oil
2 drops cinnamon essential oil
1 drop juniper essential oil

Directions

Combine all ingredients in a dark colored glass bottle (amber is best to keep light out). To use, apply one drop to your scalp, and massage into the skin before bedtime. Do this once daily.

Jasmine Perfume

Materials

4 drops jasmine essential oil

2 drops lemon essential oil

Directions

Follow the instructions in the "How to Make Your Own Perfumes Using Essential Oils" section of this book.

Woodsy Perfume

Materials

1 drop geranium essential oil
3 drops Melissa essential oil

2 drops sandalwood essential oil
1 drop basil essential oil

Directions

Follow the instructions in the "How to Make Your Own Perfumes Using Essential Oils" section of this book.

Rose Moisturizer

Materials

3 tbsp rice bran oil
1 tbsp rosehip oil
2 tsp avocado oil
3 tbsp rosewater

½ C vegetable glycerin
7 drops rose essential oil
5 drops rosewood essential oil

Directions

Combine all of the ingredients together in a glass bowl, and blend with an electric mixer until the mixture begins to thicken. Pour into a glass jar, cover, and label with the date.

Lavender Lip Balm

Materials

3 tbsp grated beeswax
1 tsp raw honey
1 tsp shea butter

4 tbsp rice bran oil
5 drops lavender essential oil

Directions

In a double boiler over medium heat, combine beeswax, honey, shea butter, and rice bran oil. When the ingredients have melted and blended together, remove from heat and stir. As mixture begins to cool, add the essential oils and continue stirring to blend. Pour into prepared lip balm tubs or tubes.

Citrus Shower Gel

Materials

8 ounces shower gel base
5 drops lemon essential oil

5 drops sweet orange essential oil
2 drops peppermint essential oil

Directions

Combine all ingredients together in a pump bottle. Shake to mix. To use, shake well and use as you would a traditional body wash.

Lavender Bubble Bath

Materials

1 C rice bran oil
½ C liquid castile soap

¼ C raw honey
5 drops lavender essential oil

Directions

Combine all of the ingredients together and pour into a pump bottle. To use, add about ¼ C of the mixture to your bathwater.

Corn and Callus Relief

Materials

2 ounces rice bran oil
12 drops lavender essential oil

5 drops myrrh essential oil

Directions

Combine all of the ingredients and store in a dark colored glass bottle (preferably amber to keep the light out). To use, shake well to mix ingredients, and apply to affected areas.

Minty-Fresh Body Powder

Materials

10 drops peppermint essential oil
5 drops spearmint essential oil

5 drops cinnamon essential oil
2 tbsp corn starch

Directions

Combine ingredients and store in a covered container. To use, apply to the skin whenever you want to feel refreshed.

ESSENTIAL OILS AND BABIES

It is important to remember that even though there are some essential oils that are good for babies, this number is limited and there are many more that should never be used in products that are for babies. This is because many of the essential oils are refreshing, which means that they are going to mess with your baby's sleeping patterns. This isn't good for the baby, and it also isn't good for you when you have to be up with them at all hours of the night because they can't sleep.

When it comes to babies and essential oils, it is important to be very careful about the oils you are using, as well as the amounts you are using. Here are some tips that will help your baby to get the most benefits from essential oils.

Limit the Amount of Oils Used – Stick with just a few essential oils, five or less, and only use the ones that are the safest, such as lavender, spearmint, sweet orange, Roman chamomile, and dill.

Lower the Dosage – Any essential oil blend used for babies must have a much lower dosage than blends for adults. A good rule of thumb is reduce the adult dosage by two thirds.

Never Put Essential Oils in Food – Babies and children should never ingest any essential oils, so if you are cooking with these oils, be sure that your little ones are eating something different. Keep all of your essential oils out of reach of children.

Always Dilute Essential Oils – When making solutions for babies, be sure to always dilute the essential oils in a carrier that is water-soluble (raw honey or vegetable glycerin are good options).

Keep Oils Away from Faces – Essential oils should never touch a baby's face, because they have extremely sensitive skin and some oils can be harsh, even when diluted.

October

BOO!!! It's time for witches, ghosts, and goblins to come around, and this month we have some delicious recipes for sweet treats (adults only as children should not ingest essential oils) to enjoy at Halloween parties. You will also find other tasty food recipes, as well as skin and hair care recipes, and a whole lot more.

Cinnamon Candy Apples

Materials

8-10 apples
8-10 popsicle sticks
2 ½ C white sugar
½ C water

½ C corn syrup
1 tbsp white vinegar
1 drop cinnamon essential oil
Red food coloring

Directions

Rinse apples and let them sit to dry. Once they are dry, insert popsicle sticks into each apple. In a saucepan over medium-low heat, combine sugar, water, corn syrup, and vinegar. Simmer, and do not stir. Heat until a candy thermometer reads 143 degrees Celsius, or 290 degrees Fahrenheit. Remove from heat, and add the cinnamon essential oil, stirring gently to mix. Dip the apples into the candy mixture, and place on a cookie sheet that has been lined with parchment paper. Let sit to harden.

Acne Steam Bath

Materials

6 drops juniper berry essential oil
3 drops cypress essential oil

5 drops lemon essential oil

Directions

Combine essential oils and extremely hot water in a glass bowl. Lean over the bowl with a towel over your head, and let the steam soak into your face. Stay like this for 5-10 minutes, and then rinse your face with cool water and pat dry.

Foot Deodorizer Powder

Materials

2 ounces talcum powder, unscented
1 tbsp baking soda
3 drops spearmint essential oil

2 drops sage essential oil
1 drop coriander essential oil

Directions

Combine all of the essential oils, and soak a cotton ball with them. Place the cotton ball in a mixture of the talcum powder and baking soda, shake, and let sit for 24-48 hours. Store in an airtight container. To use, sprinkle powder onto your feet, and in your shoes.

Skin Care Massage Oil October 4

Materials

8 drops sandalwood essential oil
8 drops rosewood essential oil

8 drops lavender essential oil
30 ml rice bran oil

Directions

Combine all of the ingredients in a glass bowl. To use, apply to any areas of your skin that need extra attention, and massage gently.

Simple Lip Balm October 5

Materials

1/3 ounce grated beeswax
3 tbsp sweet almond oil
2 tbsp macadamia nut oil

4 tsp rice bran oil
2 vitamin E capsules
5 drops peppermint essential oil

Directions

In a double boiler over medium heat, combine beeswax, almond oil, macadamia nut oil, and rice bran oil. When ingredients melt and blend together, remove from heat and stir in peppermint essential oil and liquid from vitamin E capsules. As mixture begins to thicken, pour into prepared lip balm tubs or tubes.

Love and Devotion Perfume October 6

Materials

2 drops patchioulli essential oil
1 drop clary sage essential oil

3 drops rose essential oil
3 drops rosewood essential oil

Directions

Follow the instructions in the "How to Make Your Own Perfumes Using Essential Oils" section of this book.

Relaxation Perfume October 7

Materials

2 drops bergamot essential oil
4 drops chamomile essential oil

3 drops lavender essential oil
2 drops marjoram essential oil

Directions

Follow the instructions in the "How to Make Your Own Perfumes Using Essential Oils" section of this book.

SUGAR SCRUB CUBES

Materials

2.5 ounces glycerin soap base
4 ounces shea butter
2 C white sugar

2 tbsp coconut oil
5-6 drops coconut essential oil

Directions

In a double boiler over medium heat, melt the glycerin soap base. Add the shea butter and coconut oil, stirring to mix. Remove from heat and add the essential oil and sugar, stirring to mix well. Press mixture into molds (cube or any shape you prefer) and let sit overnight in the refrigerator until solid.

CRANBERRY LIP BALM

Materials

3 tbsp grated beeswax
10-12 fresh cranberries, whole
1 tsp raw honey

1 tsp rice bran oil
1 vitamin E capsule
1 drop cranberry seed essential oil

Directions

In a double boiler over medium heat, melt the beeswax. In a glass bowl, combine cranberries, honey, and rice bran oil. Heat to boiling in the microwave, stir to blend, and strain mixture through a sieve to get rid of the cranberry skins. Add cranberry mixture to beeswax. Remove from heat and add the liquid from the vitamin E capsule and the cranberry seed essential oil. Stir with a whisk. As the mixture begins to thicken, pour into prepared lip balm tubs or tubes.

CRANBERRY HAIR RINSE

Materials

½ C fresh cranberries
½ C pureed carrots

2 tbsp lemon juice
1 drop cranberry seed essential oil

Directions

In a saucepan over medium heat, cook cranberries with a bit of water until the cranberries are soft. Mash the cranberries into a paste, straining through a sieve to remove the skins. Mix the mashed cranberries with the pureed carrots, lemon juice, and cranberry seed essential oil to create a paste. To use, apply to dry hair and wrap with plastic to seal in the warmth (take a hot bath and let the steam make this rinse work even better). Sit for 10 minutes, then rinse with clear water and use conditioner as normal. This is great for redheads to bring out the various color tones.

Cinnamon Spice Lip Gloss

Materials

1 tbsp grated beeswax
1 tsp coconut oil

1 vitamin E capsule
1-2 drops cinnamon essential oil

Directions

In a double boiler over medium heat, combine the beeswax and coconut oil. When the ingredients have melted and blended together, remove from heat and add the liquid from the vitamin E capsule and the cinnamon essential oil. Stir with a whisk, and pour into prepared lip gloss tubs.

Anti-Wrinkle Serum

Materials

2 tbsp extra virgin olive oil

10 drops geranium essential oil

Directions

Combine ingredients in a glass bowl. Pour into a dark colored glass bottle (amber is best to keep light from getting in) and store in a dark place. To use, massage a few drops into the skin on your face and neck each night.

Anti-Wrinkle Facial Mask

Materials

2 tbsp green clay

2 drops rosemary essential oil

Directions

Combine ingredients with just enough water to create a thick paste. Spread on your face and neck, and let sit for 30 minutes. Rinse with cool water. For best results, do this two to three times weekly.

Cranberry Face Wash

Materials

½ C boiling water
½ C fresh cranberries

1 tbsp dried, crushed savory leaves
1 drop cranberry seed essential oil

Directions

Puree cranberries, strain, and set aside the juice. In another bowl or cup, steep savory in boiling water for 10-15 minutes and strain. Combine both mixtures and stir to mix well. To use, soak cotton balls or pads with the mixture, and set on your face for up to 5 minutes. Remove, and rinse with clear, warm water.

Wrinkle Cream

Materials

1 tbsp cocoa butter
2 tbsp jojoba oil
1 tbsp grapefruit seed oil

1 tbsp aloe vera gel
2 drops geranium essential oil

Directions

In a double boiler over medium heat, combine cocoa butter, jojoba oil, and grapefruit seed oil. When ingredients have melted and blended together, remove from heat and add the aloe vera gel and geranium essential oil. Pour into a glass container, cover, and label with date.

Honey Cashew Candy

Materials

1 C raw honey
¼ C cashew butter

1-2 drops vanilla essential oil

Directions

In a saucepan, heat honey over medium heat until it begins to boil. Let it boil until it reaches 300 degrees F on a candy thermometer (hard crack stage). Remove from heat, add cashew butter and vanilla essential oil. Pour mixture onto a cookie sheet that has been lined with parchment paper. Allow candy to cool in the refrigerator overnight. Break into pieces and store in an airtight container in the freezer.

Cinnamon Candy Popcorn Balls

Materials

10-12 C popped popcorn
1 C white sugar
1/3 C red heart cinnamon candies
2/3 C water

1 tbsp vinegar
¼ tsp salt
1 drop cinnamon essential oil

Directions

Pop the popcorn, and remove any unpopped kernels. Place the popcorn in a greased baking pan, and place in an oven on low heat to keep it warm. Cover the sides of a heavy saucepan in butter. In the saucepan, combine sugar, water, cinnamon candies, vinegar, and salt. Bring to a boil, stirring constantly. Cook until the mixture reaches 270 degrees F on a candy thermometer (hard-ball stage). Remove from heat and add cinnamon essential oil (do not add if serving this to children). Pour over popcorn, stirring to make sure that all of the popcorn is coated. Let mixture sit for a few minutes to cool, and then form into balls.

Peppermint Foot Cream

Materials

1 ounce cocoa butter
4 ounces shea butter
1.5 ounces rice bran oil

1 ounce peppermint essential oil
¼ ounce tea tree oil
1 ounce arrowroot powder

Directions

In a double boiler over medium heat, combine cocoa butter, shea butter, and rice bran oil. Once the ingredients have melted and blended together, remove from heat and add the arrowroot powder and essential oils. Stir with a whisk to blend well. Pour into a jar, cover, label, and place in the refrigerator until mixture has become solid.

Romantic Lubricant

Materials

2 tbsp grated beeswax
1/3 C coconut oil

2 drops rose essential oil

Directions

In a double boiler over medium heat, combine the beeswax and coconut oil. When ingredients have melted and blended together, remove from heat and add the rose essential oil. Allow to cool until it has hardened. When the mixture has hardened, whip it until it is fluffy. Store in a covered glass jar for up to one year.

Mystical Body Spray

Materials

3 ounces witch hazel
1 tbsp grapefruit seed oil
3 drops lavender essential oil

3 drops neroli essential oil
3 drops spearmint essential oil

Directions

Combine all of the ingredients in a spray bottle. Shake well, label with the date, and store in the refrigerator. Shake well before each use to mix the ingredients.

Eastern Essence Perfume

Materials

3 drops jasmine essential oil
2 drops neroli essential oil

5 drops orange essential oil

Directions

Follow the instructions in the "How to Make Your Own Perfumes Using Essential Oils" section of this book.

CITRUS SCRUB   October 22

Materials

½ C coarse sea salt
½ C extra virgin olive oil

2 drops lemon essential oil
2 drops orange essential oil

Directions

Combine all ingredients in a glass bowl, mixing well to make sure that everything is well blended. Pour into glass jars, and store in a cool, dark place. To use, add about ¼ C of the salts to your bathwater.

CINNAMON/ORANGE DIFFUSER BLEND   October 23

Materials

3 drops cinnamon essential oil

5 drops sweet orange essential oil

Directions

Follow the instructions in the "Using Aroma Therapy Diffusers" section of this book.

EXCITEMENT PERFUME   October 24

Materials

4 drops Melissa essential oil
3 drops rose essential oil

1 drop jasmine essential oil
2 drops ylang ylang essential oil

Directions

Follow the instructions in the "How to Make Your Own Perfumes Using Essential Oils" section of this book.

GINGER SKIN SCRUB   October 25

Materials

3-4" chunk of fresh ginger, thinly sliced
1 C white sugar
1 C sunflower oil
3 drops ginger essential oil

Directions

In a saucepan over medium heat, combine ginger slices with just enough water to cover, and let simmer for 2-3 hours, adding water whenever necessary to keep ginger from burning to the bottom of the saucepan. Allow this ginger extract to cool. In a glass bowl, combine sugar, sunflower oil, ginger extract, and ginger essential oil, mixing well. Transfer mixture to airtight containers, and label with the date.

ORANGE/CLOVE SOAP   October 26

Materials

12 ounces glycerin soap base
1 ounce liquid aloe vera
2 vitamin E capsules
3 drops orange essential oil

1 drop clove essential oil
3-4 drops orange food-grade colorant, or
a mixture of red and yellow (optional)

Directions

In a double boiler over medium heat, melt the soap base. Remove from heat, and add aloe vera, liquid from the vitamin E capsules, essential oils, and coloring. Pour into 3-ounce soap bar molds and let sit to harden.

LIFT ME UP PERFUME   October 27

Materials

1 drop frankincense essential oil
5 drops grapefruit essential oil

2 drops rosemary essential oil
1 drop spearmint essential oil

Directions

Follow the instructions in the "How to Make Your Own Perfumes Using Essential Oils" section of this book.

CINNAMON HOT CHOCOLATE   October 28

Materials

2 tbsp cocoa
2 tbsp white sugar
1 drop cinnamon essential oil

½ C milk
½ C water

Directions

In a saucepan over medium heat, combine milk, water, cocoa, and sugar. Heat to a rolling boil. Remove from heat, and add the cinnamon essential oil. Serve with a cinnamon stick and shaved chocolate.

CINNAMON ORANGE DIFFUSER BLEND

Materials

2 drops cinnamon essential oil

4 drops orange essential oil

Directions

Follow the instructions in the "Using Aroma Therapy Diffusers" in this book.

LAVENDER BODY SPRAY

Materials

4 ounces witch hazel
1 ounce grapeseed oil

3 drops lavender essential oil
1 drop rose essential oil

Directions

Combine all ingredients in a spray bottle, and shake well to mix. Store in the refrigerator for up to one month. To use, spritz all over your body after a bath or shower.

PUMPKIN SPICE SOAP

Materials

12 ounces glycerin soap base
1 ounce liquid aloe vera

4-5 drops pumpkin seed essential oil
1 drop ginger essential oil

Directions

In a double boiler over medium heat, melt the soap base. Add the aloe vera, and remove from heat. Add the essential oils, and pour into 3-ounce soap bar molds. Allow to cool and harden.

How to Give an Essential Oil Hand Massage

Whether you want to do this at an essential oils spa party, or you just want to be able to pamper yourself whenever you want, it is nice to know how to give an essential oil hand massage. This is extremely relaxing, and if you know how to use pressure points, you can actually use these massages to treat a number of health conditions. Hand massages are easy, and you don't need to have a lot of special supplies.

Supplies You will Need

The most important thing you will need for hand massages is essential oil. There are various oils you can use, depending on the results you want. If you are looking for something that is relaxing and soothing, lavender is always a good choice. If you want to feel a bit of a tingle, try adding some peppermint essential oil. You will also need to have plenty of clean, warm towels, and a basin of warm water for rinsing. Other items you will need include grapeseed oil and coarse sea salt or Epsom salts. Once you have all of the items together, follow these steps for a relaxing hand massage.

Mix essential oils with carrier oil such as grapeseed oil. Add a couple of drops of oil for every 3-4 ounces of oil. If you are using a specific recipe, do not increase or decrease the amount of essential oils as they are recommended for a purpose. Some oils can cause sun sensitivity, and it is best to avoid being in the sun for at least 6 hours after using them on your skin. These include lemon, ginger, orange, and bergamot essential oils.

Once oils are mixed with the carrier oil, mix a few drops of the mixture with some of the coarse salt. Begin massaging this mixture onto the hands, starting at the fingertips and working your way down to the palms of your hands. If you are into using pressure points, pay close attention to the points are used for treating various problems. Rinse hands with warm water and pat dry with a clean towel.

November

With Thanksgiving being this month, it goes without saying that you are going to find some awesome pumpkin-themed recipes. There are also loads of recipes that use nutmeg and clove essential oils, for skin care and much more. Also included this month are recipes for bath products, as well as recipes for more perfumes and aroma therapy.

𝒫UMPKIN PIE SPICE OIL

Materials

30 drops cinnamon bark essential oil
30 drops ginger essential oil
30 drops nutmeg essential oil

15 drops clove essential oil
5 drops orange essential oil

Directions

Combine all ingredients together in a dark colored glass bottle (amber is best to keep light out). Use in your favorite pumpkin recipes instead of regular pumpkin spice.

𝒫UMPKIN SPICE DIFFUSER BLEND

Materials

2 drops ginger essential oil
1 drop clove essential oil

2 drops nutmeg essential oil
1 drop cinnamon essential oil

Directions

Follow the instructions in the "Using Aroma Therapy Diffusers" section of this book.

𝒜LLERGY FORMULA

Materials

30 drops lavender essential oil
30 drops lemon essential oil

30 drops peppermint essential oil
10 Empty gel caps

Directions

Combine all of the essential oils, and put inside the gel caps. Take one capsule, three times daily.

𝐻AIRSPRAY

Materials

2 tsp white sugar
½ C pure distilled water

2 drops alcohol
2 drops sweet orange essential oil

Directions

In a saucepan over medium heat, combine sugar and distilled water. Boil until sugar is dissolved, remove from heat and allow to cool. Add the alcohol and orange essential oil, and pour mixture into a mist bottle. Label with the date.

SPIRIT-LIFTING PERFUME

Materials

3 drops bergamot essential oil
2 drops jasmine essential oil

5 drops lemongrass essential oil
1 drop neroli essential oil

Directions

Follow the instructions in the "How to Make Your Own Perfumes Using Essential Oils" section of this book.

VAPOR RUB

Materials

½ C extra virgin olive oil
1 C coconut oil
¾ C grated beeswax
30 drops eucalyptus essential oil

35 drops peppermint essential oil
10 drops lavender essential oil
10 drops rosemary essential oil

Directions

In a double boiler over medium heat, combine beeswax, olive oil, and coconut oil. When ingredients have melted and blended together, remove from heat and add the essential oils. Pour into glass jars, cover, and label with the date.

HONEY LOTION BARS

Materials

2 ounces grated beeswax
1 ½ tbsp. raw honey
2 ounces shea butter

2 ounces coconut oil
1 tbsp extra virgin olive oil
5-6 drops sweet orange essential oil

Directions

In a double boiler over medium heat, combine beeswax, shea butter, and coconut oil. When ingredients have melted and blended together, remove from heat and add the olive oil, honey, and sweet orange essential oil. Pour into molds and let harden for a few hours.

HAPPINESS PERFUME

Materials

2 drops geranium essential oil
2 drops Melissa essential oil

1 drop jasmine essential oil
2 drops basil essential oil

1 drop sandalwood essential oil

Directions

Follow the instructions in the "Using Aroma Therapy Diffusers" section of this book.

PEPPERMINT BODY BUTTER

Materials

½ C coconut oil
1 C cocoa butter
½ C sweet almond oil

2 vitamin E capsules
3 drops peppermint essential oil

Directions

In a double boiler over medium heat, combine coconut oil and cocoa butter. When ingredients melt and blend together, remove from heat. Add the sweet almond oil, liquid from the vitamin E capsules, and peppermint essential oil, and mix well. Chill in the refrigerator until hardened. Whip mixture until it is light and fluffy. Pour into glass jars, cover, and label with the date.

SPICY AIR FRESHENER

Materials

4 ounces pure distilled water
25 drops marjoram essential oil
25 drops sage essential oil

30 drops clove essential oil
20 drops spearmint essential oil

Directions

Combine all ingredients together in a spray bottle. To use, spray into the air in any room in your home for a spicy scent.

PUMPKIN SOUP

Materials

2 tbsp butter
1 onion, minced
3 C vegetable broth
1 can pumpkin
1 tbsp flour

1 ½ C milk
1 tbsp raw honey
1 drop cinnamon essential oil
1 drop nutmeg essential oil
Salt and pepper to taste

Directions

Sautee onions in butter in a saucepan until soft and tender. Add flour and stir until smooth. Slowly add broth, pumpkin, honey, salt, and pepper. Bring to a boil, and reduce heat to simmer for 5-10 minutes. Add milk and heat. Add essential oils, allow to simmer for one minute, and serve.

PUMPKIN BREAD

Materials

3 C sugar
1 C vegetable oil
4 eggs, slightly beaten
1 can pumpkin (16 ounces)
3 ½ C flour

2 tsp salt
1 tsp baking soda
1 tsp baking powder
5-6 drops Pumpkin Spice Oil
2/3 C water

Directions

Preheat oven to 350 degrees. Prepare 2 loaf pans. In one bowl, combine sugar, oil, eggs, and pumpkin. In another bowl, combine the dry ingredients. Combine both mixtures with water. Pour into loaf pans, and bake for 30-40 minutes or until a toothpick inserted comes out clean.

BRONZING BODY BUTTER

Materials

1 C shea butter
½ C coconut oil
½ C extra virgin olive oil

2 tbsp cocoa
2 vitamin E capsules
6 drops peppermint essential oil

Directions

In a double boiler over medium heat, combine the shea butter and cocoa butter. When they are melted and blended together, remove from heat and let sit for a half an hour. Next, add the olive oil, cocoa, liquid from the vitamin E capsules, and the peppermint essential oil. Place in the refrigerator to allow the mixture to become firm. Then, whip the mixture with an electric mixer to make it nice and fluffy. Place in a jar, cover, and label with the date.

HAPPINESS PERFUME

Materials

4 drops neroli essential oil
1 drop patchouli essential oil

4 drops rose essential oil

Directions

Follow the instructions in the "How to Make Your Own Perfumes Using Essential Oils" section of this book.

HOLIDAY SPICE ROOM SPRAY

November 15

Materials

4 ounces pure distilled water
8-10 drops Pumpkin Spice Oil (November 1)

Directions

Combine the ingredients in a spray bottle, and shake well to make sure everything is well blended. To use, shake, and spray wherever you want a holiday pumpkin spice scent. This is a great kitchen and dining room spray for the holidays.

CITRUS MINT LAYERED SOAP

November 16

Materials

12 ounces glycerin soap base
Green and yellow food-based colorant
4 tsp liquid aloe vera

3 drops lemon essential oil
3 drops peppermint essential oil

Directions

In two double boilers over medium heat, melt half of the glycerin soap base with 2 tsp of the aloe vera in each pot. Remove both pots from heat, and in one, add the peppermint essential oil and green coloring. In the other pot, add the lemon essential oil and yellow coloring. Next, pour a half inch layer of green mixture in a small bread pan. Give it a few minutes to set, and pour a layer of yellow on. Keep repeating the process with both colors until it is all used. You may need to re-melt the soaps between layers. Let set, remove from pan, and cut into soap bars.

SOFTENING LIP BALM

November 17

Materials

3 tbsp grated beeswax
1 tsp rice bran oil
1 tsp liquid aloe vera

1 vitamin E capsule
2 drops lavender essential oil

Directions

In a double boiler over medium heat, combine beeswax, rice bran oil, and aloe vera. When the ingredients have melted and blended together, remove from heat. Add the liquid from the vitamin E capsule and the lavender essential oil. Stir with a whisk, and pour into prepared lip balm tubs or tubes.

Cinnamon Spice Tea

Materials

1 C boiling water
1 green tea bag

1 drop cinnamon essential oil
1 drop nutmeg essential oil

Directions

Steep the green tea bag in the boiling water for 10 minutes. Add the essential oils, steep for another minute or so, and remove the tea bag. Enjoy.

Minty Bath Salts

Materials

1 C Epsom salts
1 C coarse sea salt
1-2 drops green or red food-grade colorant

5 drops peppermint essential oil (or more, depending on how strong you like the scent to be)

Directions

Combine all of the ingredients together in a glass bowl. Mix well to distribute the colorant and essential oils. Store in an airtight container. To use, add a quarter cup of the mixture to your bathwater.

Healing Gel for Rashes

Materials

2 C golden flax seeds
2 C pure distilled water

¼ C liquid aloe vera
2 drops peppermint essential oil

Directions

In a saucepan over medium heat, combine flax seeds, distilled water, and aloe vera. Boil until mixture reduces to a thin, jelly-like consistency. Remove from heat and add the peppermint essential oil. Strain the flax seeds out of the mixture (this takes a while so be patient), and pour mixture into jars. Store in the refrigerator. To use, apply a small amount to rashes, burns, etc. This can also be used as a hair gel. Simply dip your comb into the gel, and then run the comb through your hair.

LIGHT AND FRESH DIFFUSER BLEND

Materials

1 drop eucalyptus essential oil
2 drops lemon essential oil
1 drop lemongrass essential oil

Directions

Follow the instructions in the "Using Aroma Therapy Diffusers" section of this book.

SOOTHING BATH OIL

Materials

½ C sweet almond oil
6 drops cedarwood essential oil

5 drops frankincense essential oil
5 drops rose essential oil

Directions

Combine all of the ingredients together in a glass bowl. To use, add three quarters of the mixture to your bathwater. After drying off, massage the remainder of the oil into your skin.

FOAMING HAND SOAP

Materials

1/3 C liquid castile soap
2/3 C pure distilled water

4 drops lemon essential oil

Directions

Combine the liquid soap and essential oil in a pump bottle, shaking gently to mix. Top up the jar with the distilled water. To use, pump out the soap, add a bit of water, and rub your hands together to create a nice lather.

PEPPERMINT SKIN TONER

Materials

1 C pure distilled water
1/3 C apple cider vinegar

60 drops peppermint essential oil

Directions

Combine all of the ingredients together in a spray bottle, shaking to blend the ingredients together. To use, shake well, and spray on your skin any time you want to feel refreshed.

Be Alert Diffuser Blend

November 25

Materials

2 drops peppermint essential oil

2 drops sweet orange essential oil

Directions

Follow the instructions in the "Using Aroma Therapy Diffusers" section of this book.

Cold and Flu Steam

November 26

Materials

3 drops tea tree essential oil
2 drops lavender essential oil

3 drops eucalyptus essential oil
2 drops peppermint essential oil

Directions

Fill a glass bowl with boiling water, and add the essential oils, stirring to mix. With a towel over your head, lean over the bowl, and let the towel cover both your head and the bowl. Inhale the steam to help clear congestion and relive other cold and flu symptoms.

Cough Relief

November 27

Materials

4 tsp rice bran oil
2 drops lavender essential oil

2 drops eucalyptus essential oil

Directions

Combine all of the ingredients together in a small glass bowl. Pour into a dark colored glass bottle (amber is best as it keeps light from affecting the quality of the essential oils). To use, apply a few drops to your throat and chest area, and massage into the skin.

Invigorating Bath Oil

November 28

Materials

½ C sweet almond oil
5 drops peppermint essential oil

2 drops pine essential oil
3 drops rosemary essential oil

Directions

Combine all of the ingredients together in a small glass bowl. To use, add three quarters of the mixture to cool bathwater to help increase your circulation. Dry off, and massage the remainder of the oil into your skin.

Coconut Body Scrub

Materials

5 tbsp Epsom salts
3 tsp coconut oil

8 drops lime essential oil
6 drops ylang ylang essential oil

Directions

Combine Epsom salts and coconut oil, stirring well to blend. Add the essential oils, and stir once again. Pour mixture into glass jars. To use, massage the mixture into your skin, being sure to get those rough patches. Make sure that you avoid your face and other sensitive areas.

Winter Warmth Perfume

Materials

3 drops ylang ylang essential oil
1 drop patchouli essential oil

2 drops black pepper essential oil
3 drops rosewood essential oil

Directions

Follow the instructions in the "How to Make Your Own Perfumes Using Essential Oils" section of this book.

THE BENEFITS OF USING ESSENTIAL OILS

There is really only one problem with essential oils, and that is that the benefits are far too numerous to list in one article. You would be surprised at the many things that essential oils can be used for. As an example, they can be used for quick pick-me-ups in aroma therapy (you can carry little vials of your favorite essential oils with you and take a whiff any time). Other benefits of using essential oils include:

Essential Oils are Organic – One of the best things about essential oils is that they are organic and completely natural. They come from the volatile liquid that is found in plants, and they can play an active role in your good health.

Essential Oils Penetrate the Skin – Unlike commercially-prepared products, essential oils will actually penetrate the skin to get to the emotional center and other parts of the brain. This is why essential oils are so great for stress relief.

Essential Oils Soothe Sore Muscles – When you rub essential oil mixtures onto your muscles, they can soothe soreness. This is especially good right after a workout.

Essential Oils are Good for Pets – Horses and dogs respond particularly well to treatments that use essential oils. The benefits are more limited for cats, but can still be used for your feline friends.

Essential Oils are Good for Your Health – There are many ways that you can use essential oils to improve your overall health. For instance, peppermint can help your digestive system.

Essential Oils are Great for House Cleaning – Instead of cleaning with chemical products, get the same results with essential oils, and breathe healthier.

Keep in mind when purchasing essential oils that they cannot be chemically reproduced. This is because they are all-natural, and it is highly unlikely that you will ever find two batches of any essential oils to be the same, but they will all have the same properties. They have multiple natural properties that make them healthy to use in many applications.

December

The holiday season is here, and it is time to start preparing your home and getting gifts ready. Home-made gifts are always loved and appreciated, so this month, we have included all kinds of fun recipes for soaps, bath salts, holiday air fresheners, and much more.

Slow Cooker Turkey Meatballs with Cranberry/BBQ Sauce

Materials

1 package ground turkey
1 C Italian bread crumbs
1 drop sage essential oil
1 drop black pepper essential oil
Salt

1 tsp garlic powder
1 tsp onion powder
1 tsp paprika
1-2 tbsp bbq sauce

Sauce

1 C bbq sauce

1 can cranberry jelly (not whole berry)

Directions

Combine ground turkey, bread crumbs, essential oils, salt, seasonings, and barbecue sauce. Mix well, and form into meatballs that are about 1 ½ inches across. In the slow cooker, combine barbecue sauce and cranberry jelly. The mixture will be lumpy at first, but as it cooks it will become nice and smooth. Add the meatballs, and cook on high for 2-3 hours. Serve over rice.

Seasonal Diffuser Blend

Materials

2 drops clove essential oil
4 drops orange essential oil

1 drop cinnamon essential oil

Directions

Follow the instructions in the "Using Aroma Therapy Diffusers" section of this book.

Citrus and Spice Hot Cider

Materials

3 C water
2 C orange juice
1 C white sugar

1 drop cinnamon essential oil
1 drop clove essential oil
Cinnamon sticks

Directions

Combine all ingredients in a saucepan and bring to a slow boil. Serve with cinnamon sticks.

GINGERBREAD MAN MINI SOAP

Materials

2-3 ounces solid glycerin soap base
1 tbsp liquid aloe vera
1 drop yellow food grade coloring

1 drop orange food grade coloring
2 drops gingerbread scent
1 drop ginger essential oil

Directions

In a double boiler over medium heat, melt the glycerin with the liquid aloe vera. When ingredients have melted together, remove from heat and add food grade coloring, gingerbread scent, and essential oil. Pour into gingerbread man chocolate molds, and let set for an hour or so. Wrap in waxed paper, or poke a hole in the top of the heads and string red ribbon through so the soaps can also be hung as scented ornaments.

SCENTED HOLIDAY ORNAMENTS

Materials

Red and green felt
Needle and thread
Polyfiber stuffing
Ruffled ribbon

Narrow ribbon for hanging
Rhinestones, glitter, and other decorations
Glue gun and hot glue
Peppermint essential oil

Directions

Cut felt into circles, bells, stars, etc. that are about 3-5 inches across. Stich half way around. Grab enough stuffing for each ornament, and add a couple of drops of peppermint essential oil to each pile of stuffing. Stuff the ornaments, and stitch closed. With the glue gun, apply the ruffled ribbon all the way around. Make a loop with the narrow ribbon, and glue it to the top of the ornament. Glue on rhinestones, glitter, and any other decorations you wish to use.

SWEET CRANBERRY SAUCE

Materials

1 package fresh cranberries
1 C water
2 C white sugar

½ C orange juice
1 drop cinnamon essential oil
1 drop clove essential oil

Directions

In a saucepan, combine water, sugar, orange juice, and cranberries. Cook over medium-low heat until cranberries begin to pop. Remove from heat, and add essential oils. Pour into a Mason jar and store in the refrigerator for up to one month.

HOLIDAY PERFUME

Materials

2 drops clove essential oil
2 drops cinnamon essential oil

2 drops orange essential oil
1 drop frankincense essential oil

Directions

Follow the instructions in the "How to Make Your Own Perfumes Using Essential Oils" section in this book.

STAR SOAP

Materials

12 ounces solid glycerin soap base
Red food grade coloring
Green food grade coloring
2 tbsp liquid aloe vera

2 vitamin E capsules
Peppermint essential oil
Star-shaped soap molds

Directions

In a double boiler over medium heat, combine half of the glycerin soap base, 1 tbsp aloe vera, and the liquid from one of the vitamin E capsules. When the glycerin has melted and the ingredients are blended together, remove from heat, add peppermint essential oil and green coloring. Pour into molds, filling them half way. When this has set, repeat the process with the red coloring, and finish filling the molds. When the soaps have completely set, remove from molds, and wrap in colorful paper with a ribbon.

STOVETOP KITCHEN FRESHENER

Materials

2 C water
2 drops cinnamon essential oil

1 drop clove essential oil
1 drop orange essential oil

Directions

Place all ingredients into a small saucepan, and simmer over medium-low heat. The scent will fill the entire kitchen, and even go throughout the rest of your home.

Holiday Bath Salts

Materials

2 C Epsom salts
2 C coarse sea salt
4 drops cinnamon essential oil
Red and green food grade coloring

Directions

Mix 1 C Epsom salts and 1 C coarse sea salt into a bowl. Add a couple of drops of red coloring and 2 drops essential oil. The mixture will be pink in color. Repeat process with the green, for pale green bath salts. In fancy bottles, layer the colors so you have strips. Cap, and tie with a pretty ribbon and bow. Label to make the gift even more personal.

Orange/Cinnamon Facial Scrub

Materials

5 tbsp almond meal
1 tsp orange zest
2 tbsp raw honey
½ tsp ground cinnamon

2 drops cinnamon essential oil
2 drops sweet orange essential oil
Plain yogurt

Directions

Combine the almond meal and orange zest in a glass bowl. Add enough yogurt to create a thick paste. Warm the honey, and add the almond meal mixture. Add ground cinnamon and essential oils, and stir to mix. To use, massage mixture onto your face and neck, and let sit for a few minutes. Rinse with warm water.

Peppermint Lip Balm

Materials

3 tbsp grated beeswax
1 tbsp rice bran oil

1 tsp liquid aloe vera
3 drops peppermint essential oil

Directions

In a double boiler over medium heat, combine beeswax, rice bran oil, and aloe vera. When the ingredients have melted and blended together, remove from heat and add essential oil. Pour into prepared lip balm tubs or tubes.

HOLIDAY DIFFUSER BLEND

Materials

3 drops pine essential oil
3 drops frankincense essential oil

2 drops sandalwood essential oil

Directions

Follow the instructions in the "Using Aroma Therapy Diffusers" section of this book.

BAKED HAM WITH GLAZE
December 14

Materials

1 large bone-in ham
1 C brown sugar
½ C vinegar
½ C orange juice

1 drop clove essential oil
Whole cloves
½ C orange marmalade
1 can pineapple rings

Directions

Preheat oven to 350 degrees. In a bowl, combine the brown sugar, vinegar, orange juice, marmalade, and juice from the pineapple. Place the ham in a roaster, and place whole cloves in the ham in a checkerboard pattern. Add a bit of water to the bottom of the roaster, and put a couple of spoonfuls of the glaze on the ham. About every ½ hour while baking, add more of the glaze, making sure to save ½ C for the end. Bake for 3-4 hours, depending on the size of the ham. In the last 15 minutes of baking, add the clove essential oil to the glaze. Pour over the ham, and finish cooking, uncovered so the glaze gets nice and sticky.

ORANGE CLOVE CLOSET FRESHENER
December 15

Materials

Large oranges
Whole cloves
Clove essential oil

Narrow ribbon
Pins with ball ends

Directions

Poke the cloves into the oranges in rows all the way around until you have them all over the oranges. Next, cut ribbon long enough to wrap around the oranges twice (all four sides), and tie into bows to use for hanging. Secure the ribbons with the pins. Add a couple of drops of clove essential oil to the ribbons.

Candy Cane Drawer Freshener

Materials

Peppermint essential oil
Lace handkerchiefs

Cotton balls
Ribbon

Directions

Place a drop or two of peppermint essential oil on each cotton ball. Place 2-3 cotton balls in the center of each handkerchief, and tie with the ribbon to create a sachet.

Scar Treatment

Materials

5 drops myrrh essential oil
5 drops helychrysm essential oil
4 drops lavender essential oil

2 drops sandalwood essential oil
1 tbsp rice bran oil

Directions

Combine all of the ingredients, and massage onto scars daily.

Invigorating Massage Oil

Materials

1 ounce extra virgin olive oil
10 drops peppermint essential oil

5 drops grapefruit essential oil

Directions

Combine all of the ingredients in a dark glass bottle (amber is a good choice because it doesn't let light in). Use as a massage oil when you need a quick pick-me-up.

Holiday Air Spray

Materials

4 ounces pure distilled water
5 ml emulsifier
20 drops sage essential oil

25 drops clove essential oil
20 drops spearmint essential oil
15 drops marjoram essential oil

Directions

Combine emulsifier and essential oils in a spray bottle, and then add the distilled water. Shake well, and allow to sit for 24 hours before using. To use, shake well, and spray around your home.

Holiday Air Spray 2

Materials

4 ounces pure distilled water
35 drops clove bud essential oil
35 drops cinnamon essential oil

20 drops ginger essential oil
20 drops sweet orange essential oil

Directions

Combine emulsifier and essential oils in a spray bottle, and then add the distilled water. Shake well, and allow to sit for 24 hours before using. To use, shake well, and spray around your home.

Lavender Face Lotion

Materials

3 ½ tbsp shea butter
2 tbsp jojoba oil

3 tbsp liquid aloe vera
4 drops lavender essential oil

Directions

In a double boiler over medium heat, melt the shea butter and jojoba oil until they are combined. Add the aloe vera, and pour mixture into a food processor and whip for 5 minutes. Add the essential oils, and pour into a jar. Cover, and label with the date. This can be stored for up to three months. Add a ribbon around the lid to make a nice holiday gift.

Candy Cane Skin Toner

Materials

¾ C pure distilled water or filtered water
¼ C apple cider vinegar

35 drops peppermint essential oil

Directions

Pour water and vinegar into a spray bottle. Add the essential oil. Mist your face as you need it, at any time of the day for a refreshing and cooling effect.

Facial Moisturizer

Materials

2 tbsp extra virgin olive oil
15 drops rose essential oi
5 drops lavender essential oil

5 drops lemon essential oil
2 drops patchouli essential oil

Directions

Mix all of the ingredients together in a small glass bowl. Apply to dampened skin and massage. Dap excess oil off your face with a tissue.

Holiday Hot Chocolate Gift Pack

Materials

1 tbsp cocoa (more or less to taste)
1 tbsp white sugar (more or less to taste)
2 drops peppermint essential oil
Small dark colored glass vial with cap
Chocolate spoon

2 small plastic bags
1 Nice Mug
Colored cellophane
Ribbon

Directions

Place the cocoa and sugar in separate small plastic bags. Put the essential oil into the vial, and make sure it is capped. Place all of the items, with the chocolate spoon, into the mug. Wrap with cellophane and tie with a ribbon.

Holiday Turkey

Materials

1 large turkey
1 large onion
2 drops sage essential oil
1 clove garlic, minced
1 C butter
Pepper

1 tsp paprika
½ tsp chili powder
1 tsp poultry seasoning
2 tbsp soya sauce
½ C orange juice

Directions

Preheat oven to 350 degrees. Mix butter, 1 drop sage essential oil, pepper, poultry seasoning, chili powder, paprika, and minced garlic. Pull back the turkey skin, and massage the meat with the butter mixture. Put about an inch of water in the roaster, and lay turkey inside. Add the onions to the water, and pour in the orange juice. Pour the soya sauce over the turkey. Bake for 4-5 hours, depending on the size of the turkey.

*B*OXING DAY LEFTOVER TURKEY STIR-FRY

Materials

2 C leftover turkey, chopped
1 C mixed frozen vegetables
2 tbsp soya sauce
1 drop ginger essential oil

1 clove garlic, crushed
1 tbsp brown sugar
½ C water

Directions

In a deep frying pan, combine water, brown sugar, soya sauce, and garlic. When the brown sugar has dissolved, add the leftover turkey and frozen vegetables. When the veggies are hot, add the essential oil and serve stir-fry over a bed of rice.

*M*INTY FRESH FLOOR CLEANER

Materials

1 gallon hot water
10 drops peppermint essential oil

10 drops eucalyptus essential oil
10 drops orange essential oil

Directions

Pour the water into a bucket, and add the essential oils. Stir to mix, and use to scrub your floors and leave a clean, fresh scent throughout your home.

*S*INK STAIN REMOVER

Materials

¼ C washing soda
¼ C baking soda

¾ C white vinegar
8 drops tea tree essential oil

Directions

Mix sodas and essential oils in a container with a lid. Shake well before each use. To use, sprinkle a little bit on the sink stain and scrub. Rinse with vinegar, followed by hot water.

KITCHEN WIPES 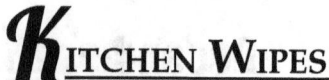 December 29

Materials

12" squares of cotton fabric
1 C water
1 ounce liquid castile soap
8 drops lemon essential oil

Directions

Combine the liquid ingredients and essential oil in a jar, cover tightly and shake to mix. Stuff as many of the fabric squares into the jar as will fit. Cover until you are ready to use. After you use a cloth, you may put it back into the jar to use again later.

MOISTURIZING FACIAL MASK December 30

Materials

1 ounce red clay
1 tsp liquid aloe vera
1 tbsp rice bran oil

1 vitamin E capsule
2 drops lavender essential oil

Directions

Combine clay, aloe vera, rice bran oil, liquid from vitamin E capsule, and lavender essential oil into a small glass bowl. To use, apply all over the face and neck, avoiding the eyes, nostrils, and mouth. Leave on for about 20 minutes, and then rinse with warm water.

NEW YEAR'S EVE PERFUME December 31

Materials

3 drops bergamot essential oil
3 drops rose essential oil

4 drops sandalwood essential oil
1 drop palmarosa essential oil

Directions

Follow the instructions in the "How to Make Your Own Perfumes Using Essential Oils" section in this book.

CONCLUSION

Dozens of hours of research has gone into compiling these recipes, so you can have hundreds of essential oil recipes for tons of different uses. You can find hundreds more recipes in books at your local library, and of course, on the Internet. The articles in this book are so you can refer to basic directions for making just about anything with essential oils, from pet care products to perfumes to skin care and so much more. We hope you have enjoyed this book, and that you will put the many recipes to good use.

Bonus Essential Oils

1NTRODUCTION

Because you loved the "365 Essential Oil Recipes for 365 Days" book, we have more great recipes for you to try. Here are an additional 45 bonus essential recipes for everything from facial care to soap to bath products and even food recipes.

POISE PERFUME

Materials

1 drop basil essential oil
3 drops bergamot essential oil

2 drops coriander essential oil
3 drops petit grain essential oil

Directions

Follow the instructions in the "How to Make Your Own Perfumes Using Essential Oils" section of the "365 Essential Oil Recipes for 365 Days" book.

RELAXATION AROMATHERAPY BLEND

Materials

2 drops benzoin essential oil
2 drops rose essential oil

2 drops verbena essential oil

Directions

Follow the instructions in the "Using Aromatherapy Diffusers" section of the "365 Essential Oil Recipes for 365 Days" book.

SKIN SOFTENING SOAP

Materials

12 ounces solid glycerin
4-5 drops lavender essential oil
2 drops rose essential oil

1 tbsp liquid aloe vera
1 vitamin E capsule
Food grade colorant

Directions

In a double boiler over medium heat, melt the glycerin with the aloe vera and the liquid from the vitamin E capsule. Remove from heat, and add the essential oils and colorant. Pour into molds and let set for a couple of hours.

DRY SHAMPOO

Materials

1 C corn starch
1 drop tea tree oil

1 drop peppermint essential oil

Directions

In a glass bowl, mix all of the ingredients. Pour into a glass jar and shake well to make sure that everything is mixed well. Store in a cool, dark place.

Citrus Air Freshener

Materials

2 C pure distilled water
3 drops sweet orange essential oil

2 drops lemon essential oil

Directions

Combine all of the ingredients together in a spray bottle. To use, spray in any room in the home. This is a great kitchen and bathroom air freshener.

Spearmint Lip Balm

Materials

3 tbsp grated beeswax
3 drops spearmint essential oil

1 tbsp rice bran oil
1 vitamin E capsule

Directions

In a double boiler over medium heat, melt the beeswax with the rice bran oil. When these ingredients have melted and blended together, remove from heat and add the liquid from the vitamin E capsule and spearmint essential oil. Pour into prepared lip balm tubs or tubes

Soothing Perfume

Materials

2 drops frankinscence essential oil
2 drops Melissa essential oil

2 drops lavender essential oil

Directions

Follow the instructions in the "How to Make Your Own Perfumes Using Essential Oils" section of the "365 Essential Oil Recipes for 365 Days" book.

Skin Softening Face Mask

Materials

1 ounce green clay
3 tbsp pure distilled water
1 tsp vegetable glycerin

1 tsp liquid aloe vera
1 drop rose essential oil
1 drop lavender essential oil

Directions

Follow the instructions in the "How to Make Clay Facial Masks with Essential Oils" section of the "365 Essential Oils Recipes for 365 Days" book.

LEMON BATH SALTS

Materials

1 C Epsom Salts
1 C coarse sea salt

4-5 drops lemon essential oil
2 drops lemongrass essential oil

Directions

In a glass bowl, combine all of the ingredients together, making sure to mix well. You can add a bit of food grade colorant if you want. Pour mixture into glass jars, cover, and label with the date.

WINTER HOLIDAY PERFUME

Materials

2 drops cinnamon essential oil
1 drops peppermint essential oil

1 drop clove essential oil

Directions

Follow the instructions in the "How to Make Your Own Perfumes Using Essential Oils" section of the "365 Essential Oil Recipes for 365 Days" book.

SWEET LEMONADE

Materials

1 C spring water
¼ C lemon juice

2-3 tbsp raw honey
1 drop lemon essential oil

Directions

Combine all of the ingredients in a tall glass, mix well, and add ice.

SUNSHINE BODY SPRAY

Materials

½ C pure distilled water
½ C witch hazel

3 drops lemon essential oil
1 drop orange essential oil

Directions

Combine all of the ingredients in a spray bottle and shake to mix. To use, shake well, and spritz all over your body.

Honey Garlic Sauce

Materials

1 C dark molasses
1 clove garlic, minced
½ C brown sugar

2 tbsp soya sauce
1 drop ginger essential oil
1 tsp powdered ginger

Directions

In a saucepan over medium heat, combine the molasses, soya sauce, brown sugar, garlic, and powdered ginger. Cook until the sugar dissolves. Remove from heat and add the ginger essential oil. Use immediately, or pour into a jar, cover, and store in the fridge for up to one week.

Tingly Facial Mask

Materials

1 ounce green clay
1 tbsp rice bran oil
2 tbsp pure distilled water

2 drops peppermint essential oil
1 drop spearmint essential oil

Directions

Follow the instructions in the "How to Make Clay Facial Masks with Essential Oils" section of the "365 Essential Oils Recipes for 365 Days" book.

After-Sun Aloe Vera Gel

Materials

5 tbsp aloe vera gel
2 drops chamomile essential oil
2 drops lavender essential oil

1 drop rose essential oil
1 drop lemongrass essential oil

Directions

In a glass bowl, combine all of the ingredients and mix well. Pour mixture into a glass bottle, cover, and label with the date. Store in the refrigerator for refreshing after-sun care.

Face Lotion

Materials

1 small cucumber
4 tbsp plain yogurt

2 drops rose essential oil
1 drop chamomile essential oil

Directions

Run the cucumber through a juicer. Combine 2 tbsp of the cucumber juice with the rest of the ingredients. Pour into a glass jar, cover, and label with the date. To use, put a small amount on your fingertips and massage into facial skin.

CHERRY LIP BALM

Materials

3 tbsp grated beeswax
1 tsp raw honey
1 tsp cocoa butter

1-2 drops cherry blossom essential oil
1-2 drops cherry lip balm flavoring

Directions

In a double boiler over medium heat, combine beeswax, raw honey, and cocoa butter. When the ingredients have melted and blended together, remove from heat and add the cherry blossom essential oil and lip balm flavoring. Pour into prepared lip balm tubes or tubs.

VALENTINE'S DAY PERFUME

Materials

2 drops frankincense essential oil
1 drop rose essential oil

1 drop lavender essential oil

Directions

Follow the instructions in the "How to Make Your Own Perfumes Using Essential Oils" section of the "365 Essential Oil Recipes for 365 Days" book.

ICED TEA

Materials

5 C spring water
2 regular tea bags
1 green tea bag

1 drop lemon essential oil
Juice from 1 lemon
Raw honey

Directions

Combine all of the ingredients together in a glass pitcher. Sweeten to taste with raw honey. Serve over ice.

Holiday Diffuser Blend

Materials

2 drops clove essential oil

1 drop cinnamon essential oil
1 drop peppermint essential oil

Directions

Follow the instructions in the "Using Aromatherapy Diffusers" section of the "365 Essential Oil Recipes for 365 Days" book.

Perfumed Body Spray

Materials

½ C pure distilled water
½ C witch hazel
2 drops bergamot essential oil

1 drop frankincense essential oil
1 drop lavender essential oil

Directions

Combine all of the ingredients in a spray bottle and store in the fridge. To use, shake well, and spray all over your body.

Scented Dryer Balls

Materials

1 small skein 100% wool yarn
lemon essential oil

Pantyhose

Directions

Unravel the yarn, and re-roll it into small balls. Put the balls inside the pantyhose, tying a knot between each ball. Wash on the hot cycle with a cold rinse, and dry on the hottest setting. This will cause the balls to "felt". You may need to do this a few times to get the felting right. To use, add a couple of drops of lemon essential oil to each ball, and place in the dryer with your laundry.

Facial Oil

Materials

2 tbsp rice bran oil
1 tbsp jojoba oil
1 tbsp rosehip oil
2 drops jasmine essential oil
2 drops sandalwood essential oil

Directions

Combine the rice bran oil, jojoba oil, and rosehip oil in a dark glass bottle (preferably amber to keep the light out). Add the essential oils and shake to mix. Cover, and label with the date.

PAPER BAG CHICKEN

Materials

1 small roaster chicken
1 tsp soya sauce
1 C butter
1 clove garlic, minced
1 small onion, minced

½ tsp cayenne pepper
½ tsp paprika
½ tsp poultry seasoning
1 drop sage essential oil
1 paper grocery bag

Directions

Preheat oven to 350 degrees. In a glass bowl, combine soya sauce, butter, garlic, onion, seasonings, and sage essential oil. Clean and dry the chicken. Pull back the skin (without removing it), and massage the meat with the butter mixture. Put skin back in place, and put the chicken into the paper bag. Fold the top of the bag over, place into a roaster, and bake in the oven (1/2 hour per pound of meat).

FOOT BATH

Materials

3 drops geranium essential oil
3 drops lemongrass essential oil

3 drops lime essential oil

Directions

Fill a foot soak basin with hot water and add the essential oils. Stir to mix, and soak feet for 10-15 minutes, or until water starts to cool down.

HAND CREAM

Materials

6 tbsp cocoa butter
1 tbsp jojoba oil
2 tbsp grated beeswax
3 tbsp rice bran oil
1 tbsp rosehip oil

10 drops geranium essential oil
5 drops Melissa essential oil
2 drops parsley essential oil
3 drops lavender essential oil

Directions

In a double boiler over medium heat, combine cocoa butter, rice bran oil, jojoba oil, and beeswax. When the ingredients have melted and blended together, remove from heat and stir. Add the essential oils, and stir until mixture begins to thicken. Pour into glass jars, cover, and label with the date.

Body Moisturizer

Materials

3 tbsp rice bran oil
1 tbsp aloe vera gel
1 tbsp carrot-infused oil

6 drops geranium essential oil
5 drops lavender essential oil
1 drop rose essential oil

Directions

In a glass bowl, combine all of the ingredients and mix with an electric beater until the mixture begins to thicken. Pour into a glass jar, cover, and label with the date.

Light Summer Perfume

Materials

2 drops lemon essential oil
2 drops lemongrass essential oil

1 drop grapefruit essential oil
2 drops sweet orange essential oil

Directions

Follow the instructions in the "How to Make Your Own Perfumes Using Essential Oils" section of the "365 Essential Oil Recipes for 365 Days" book.

Facial Toner

Materials

½ C pure distilled water
½ C rosewater
2 drops chamomile essential oil

1 drop geranium essential oil
3 drops rose essential oil

Directions

Mix all of the ingredients together in a dark colored glass bottle (amber is best as it prevents light from getting in). Cover and label with the date, and shake well before each use to blend the ingredients.

Cleansing Cream

Materials

1 tbsp grated beeswax
½ C rice bran oil
1 tbsp pure distilled water
2 drops frankincense essential oil
2 drops lavender essential oil
2 drops neroli essential oil

Directions

In a double boiler over medium heat, combine beeswax and rice bran oil. Heat the distilled water in another double boiler. When the ingredients have melted and blended together, add the warmed water drop by drop, stirring with a whisk. As the mixture begins to thicken, add the essential oils. Pour into glass jars, cover, and label with the date.

KIDS' SOAP

Materials

12 ounces solid glycerin
1 tbsp aloe vera gel
3-4 drops lemon essential oil

Food grade colorant
Small toys (from gumball machines)

Directions

In a double boiler over medium heat, melt the glycerin. Add the aloe vera. Remove from heat, and add the essential oils and colorant. Fill soap molds half way with the mixture, and let set. When it is set, place a toy on top of each bit of hardened soap. Re-melt the rest of the mixture, and pour on top of the toy and allow to set for a few hours.

RASPBERRY LIP BALM

Materials

3 tbsp grated beeswax
1 tsp liquid aloe vera
1 tbsp rice bran oil

1 tsp raw honey
2 drops raspberry essential oil
1-2 drops raspberry lip balm flavoring

Directions

In a double boiler over medium heat, combine beeswax and rice bran oil. When ingredients have melted and blended together, remove from heat and add the aloe vera, raspberry essential oil, and raspberry lip balm flavoring. Pour into prepared lip balm tubs or tubes and let set.

SWEET ORANGE BATH SALTS

Materials

1 C Epsom salt
1 C coarse sea salt

3 drops sweet orange essential oil
2-3 drops orange food grade colorant

Directions

In a glass bowl, combine all of the ingredients and mix well. Pour into glass jars, cover, and label with the date. To use, pour ¼ C of the mixture into your bathwater.

Refreshing Perfume

Materials

2 drops grapefruit essential oil
2 drops orange essential oil
1 drop lavender essential oil

1 drop rose essential oil
1 drop lemongrass essential oil

Directions

Follow the instructions in the "How to Make Your Own Perfumes Using Essential Oils" section of the "365 Essential Oil Recipes for 365 Days" book.

Festive Diffuser Blend

Materials

2 drops sandalwood essential oil
2 drops cinnamon essential oil

1 drop frankincense essential oil
1 drop basil essential oil

Directions

Follow the instructions in the "Using Aromatherapy Diffusers" section of the "365 Essential Oil Recipes for 365 Days" book.

Office Diffuser Blend

Materials

2 drops bergamot essential oil
3 drops jasmine essential oil

1 drop Ylang Ylang essential oil

Directions

Follow the instructions in the "Using Aromatherapy Diffusers" section of the "365 Essential Oil Recipes for 365 Days" book.

Healing Bath Fizz

Materials

1 C baking soda
½ C citric acid
2 tbsp rice bran oil
8 drops chamomile essential oil
5 drops geranium essential oil
4 drops verbena essential oil

Directions

In a glass bowl, combine the baking soda and citric acid. Add the rice bran oil and essential oils, and mix thoroughly. Scoop mixture into molds and pack tightly. Let sit overnight, remove from molds, and store in an airtight container. To use, place 1-2 pieces in your bathwater.

DRY SKIN FACIAL MASK

Materials

2 ounces green clay
3 tsp corn flour
1 egg yolk

2 drops carrot essential oil
1 drop evening primrose essential oil
1 tsp pure distilled water

Directions

Follow the instructions in the "How to Make Clay Facial Masks with Essential Oils" section of the "365 Essential Oils Recipes for 365 Days" book.

SORE THROAT REMEDY

Materials

1 C boiling spring water
1 tbsp raw honey
2 tbsp lemon juice

1 drop lemon essential oil
1 drop ginger essential oil

Directions

Combine all of the ingredients in a mug, and stir well. Drink while mixture is steaming for best results.

HOUSEHOLD CLEANING SPRAY

Materials

2 C pure distilled water
2 C white vinegar

10 drops lemon essential oil
5 drops pine essential oil

Directions

Combine ingredients in a spray bottle and shake well to mix. To use, shake well, and spray on surfaces that need cleaning. This can also be used as a floor cleaner, and is great for hardwood floors.

$\mathcal{A}$CHING MUSCLE MASSAGE OIL

Materials

5 ounces rice bran oil
4 drops peppermint essential oil
4 drops thyme essential oil

4 drops lavender essential oil
2 drops marjoram essential oil

Directions

In a glass bowl, combine all of the ingredients and stir well to blend. Pour into a dark colored glass bottle (preferably amber to keep light from getting in). To use, apply a couple of drops of the mixture to the affected are and massage into skin.

$\mathcal{L}$IGHT AIR FRESHENER

Materials

2 ounces pure distilled water
15 drops lavender essential oil
10 drops sweet orange essential oil

10 drops lemon essential oil
10 drops grapefruit essential oil
5 drops lime essential oil

Directions

Combine all of the ingredients in a spray bottle. Shake well before each use.

$\mathcal{A}$LOE VERA SOAP

Materials

12 ounces solid glycerin
3 tbsp liquid aloe vera

1 vitamin E capsule
4 drops lavender essential oil

Directions

In a double boiler over medium heat, melt the glycerin. Remove from heat, and add the aloe vera, liquid from the vitamin E capsule, and lavender essential oil. Pour into soap molds and allow mixture to set.

$\mathcal{O}$RANGE CRANBERRY CHOCOLATE BARK

Materials

1 bag semi-sweet chocolate chips
½ C chopped nuts
½ C dried cranberries
½ tsp orange extract
1 drop orange essential oil
¼ ounce paraffin wax (optional)

Directions

In a double boiler over medium heat, melt the chocolate chips. You may add a bit of paraffin wax to make the chocolate shiny (it also helps to keep the chocolate from melting in your hands when you are eating). Remove from heat, and stir in the orange extract, orange essential oil, nuts, and dried cranberries. Pour mixture onto a baking sheet that has been lined with parchment paper. When mixture has set, break into pieces and store in an airtight container in the fridge for up to two weeks.

Anxiety Relief for Small Dogs

Materials

2 tbsp liquid aloe vera
2 drops frankincense essential oil

2 drops lavender essential oil
1 drop Ylang Ylang essential oil

Directions

Combine the ingredients in a dark colored glass bottle (amber is best for keeping light out). Cover and label with the date. To use, shake well, place a small amount on your hands, and apply to the bottom of your dog's neck.

CONCLUSION

We hope you have enjoyed these additional 45 essential oils recipes. Once you get used to using essential oils, feel free to change up any of these recipes to make your own special blends for skin and hair care, general health, house cleaning, and a whole lot more.